SPITTING

Helen Bynum is a freelance historian and author of *Tropical Medicine in the 20th Century*. Together with William Bynum, she has written *Remarkable Plants* (2014) and edited *Great Discoveries in Medicine* (2011) and the award winning *Dictionary of Medical Biography* (5 vols).

SPITTING BLOOD

The History of Tuberculosis

HELEN BYNUM

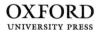

OXFORD
UNIVERSITY PRESS

OXFORD
UNIVERSITY PRESS

Great Clarendon Street, Oxford, OX2 6DP,
United Kingdom

Oxford University Press is a department of the University of Oxford.
It furthers the University's objective of excellence in research, scholarship,
and education by publishing worldwide. Oxford is a registered trade mark of
Oxford University Press in the UK and in certain other countries

First published 2012
First published in paperback 2015

Impression: 1

Published in the United States of America by Oxford University Press
198 Madison Avenue, New York, NY 10016, United States of America

British Library Cataloguing in Publication Data

Data available

ISBN 978–0–19–954205–5 (Hbk.)
ISBN 978–0–19–872751–4 (Pbk.)

Printed and bound in Great Britain by
Clays Ltd, St Ives plc

For Bill
ne plus ultra

ACKNOWLEDGEMENTS

The team at OUP—Latha and Emma in particular—deserve great thanks for encouraging the Biographies of Disease series, in which this book started life. They have proven to be incredibly patient too. Jenny Lunsford's production management has been superb. Jacqueline Harvey (copy-editor) and Andrew Hawkey (proof-reader) have helped save my blushes. Alasdair McCartney at Wellcome Images provided a wonderfully efficient service. I am grateful to the Orwell Archive at UCL Special Collections for help with Orwell's medical records.

Jonathan Bynum very kindly acted as postman when a book purchase had gone astray—thank you, there's nothing quite like help at the eleventh hour. Andrew Jones posted me his copy of *The Constant Gardener*, quicker and much nicer than Amazon. Sally Sheard and Sarah Duignan are never more than an email away.

Thanks also to all those people who asked me how the book was progressing and mentioned in passing their personal brush with tuberculosis. It reminded me sharply how common the disease had been and how people had suffered. Janet Fisher's 'Burial Book'—the handwritten records of Branch 315 of the Rational Sick and Burial Association—is a piece of her family archive. The frequent references to death from phthisis in the late 19th and early 20th century in rural Suffolk made for plain reading.

At the start two anonymous readers commented very helpfully on the proposed outline of the book for the press. At the end Clark Lawlor read an early draft and Mick Worboys, having provided inspiration through his own work on tuberculosis, came up with extremely helpful observations on the shaping of the final draft. I am grateful to him. And to all those others whose work I have benefited from reading, many of which appear in the Further Reading at the end. My mistakes are my own, of course.

I simply couldn't do any of this without Bill. He is all. He only complained a bit when we had to go through the day's reading or writing, one more time over dinner, every night.

CONTENTS

LIST OF ILLUSTRATIONS

PROLOGUE

George Orwell (1903–1950)

It's impossible to know exactly when the writer George Orwell contracted pulmonary tuberculosis. At some point he was sufficiently exposed to the *Mycobacterium tuberculosis* (the most common of the family of mycobacteria that cause this disease) for these organisms to take up residence in his body. In Orwell's case, as with the majority of those who suffer from tuberculosis, the bacteria lodged in his lungs. If they had been contained there by the immune system, he might have experienced some slight symptoms, passed off as a cold or flu, or nothing at all. And that could have been the end of the story.

Had the bacteria remained trapped in a calcified nodule or tubercle, the life of one of the leading leftist writers of the late 1930s would probably have been quite different. Instead he emerged from popular obscurity to public success with *Animal Farm* (published on 17 August 1945, two days after Japan surrendered) in mediocre health, which he had endured with considerable stoicism or at least studied indifference. Rather than 1984 being his 'last great work'—a description he neither subscribed to nor intended—he might at the very least have gone on to complete the next novel already sketched in his mind, besides producing more of his insightful, elegant reviews and essays. Effectively a bed-bound invalid, he lived a mere seven severely compromised months after the publication (on 8 June 1949) of his chilling book. Some of the details of 1984—the appearance of the central character, Winston Smith—may be based on his own experiences of suffering. Aware of the bitter irony—'I've made all this money, and now I'm going to die'—he drowned in his own blood after a severe lung haemorrhage on 21 January 1950, aged 46, leaving a widow and an adopted son just under 5 years old.[1]

As a victim of tuberculosis Orwell died from one of the oldest of human diseases. 'Tuberculosis' is an easy shorthand for pulmonary tuberculosis, from which most of the tuberculous suffer, although the disease is horribly ubiquitous; besides the lungs it destroys the tissues of most of the body's systems—central nervous, circulatory, lymphatic, gastrointestinal, genitourinary as well as the bones, joints, and skin. Something of an oddity among the infectious diseases, tuberculosis has an undefined incubation period (from contact to symptoms), and a typically chronic course. Tuberculosis can be a quick killer, especially in its meningeal form in the brain, but usually it isn't. It carries out its destructive tendencies over a much longer period, often as the body's own defences wane. The risk of contracting tuberculosis, and its progress over time, are heavily dependent on the health of the victims and the conditions in which they live. It is among the best examples of a disease with a complex multi-factorial causation. Ghastly as its individual effects are, these were cruelly magnified as sustained epidemic phases flared around the world: since everything about tuberculosis is chronic, its epidemics last much longer than epidemics of other infectious diseases. When the problems the disease posed were bad enough at a national level, or at least gained sufficient recognition, responses to tuberculosis drove social and political change.

The infant Eric Blair (Orwell adopted his pen-name in 1932) was reputed to be a 'chesty' baby and child whose chronic cough and 'wheeziness' drew comment from neighbours and teachers. Photographs show a round-faced boy and adolescent. He was active enough not to be carrying 'puppy fat', nor was he prevented from swimming and playing the 'wall game' at Eton because of his lungs. After Eton, George went out to Burma as a member of the Indian Imperial Police. Five years of empire was enough for this would-be socialist. In 1927 he returned home on sick leave, diagnosed with dengue-fever, resigned the service, and began a new career as a writer.

For the rest of his life Orwell had a more or less peripatetic existence. In the late 1920s and 1930s this was sometimes for its research potential. 'Going native' in his own country as a tramp involved sleeping rough, in 'the spike' (the casual ward of the poorhouse), or the very cheapest public lodging houses. By seeing and doing he learned what it was like to pick hops in Kent; wash dishes in Paris; teach prep-school kids in Middlesex; sell second-hand books in Hampstead; live on the dole or less in the depressed areas of northern England or, if lucky, work down a mine there; keep shop; tend a garden and goat in Hertfordshire; and fight and be injured by the Fascists in Spain. Always he was writing—fiction, a little poetry, reviews, essays—and trying to live on the minimum earned income so there would be more time at the typewriter. Orwell's long-standing lung troubles continued through his adventures. No winter would be complete without an attack of bronchitis. Of four bouts of pneumonia, two led to hospitalization, Paris in 1929 and Uxbridge in 1933. The chronic cough persisted, but then he smoked all the time too. Lots of people coughed and smoked.

In early March 1938 Orwell was at home in Wallington, Hertfordshire. He had recovered from the rigours of the Spanish Civil War the year before, including a gunshot wound through the throat. The manuscript of *Homage to Catalonia* had been finished at the end of January and he was indulging in his favourite hobby—growing vegetables—although this necessitated paid help with the heavy digging. His cough turned nasty—'I've been spitting blood again, it always turns out not to be serious, but it's alarming when it happens.'[2] If this was a frequent occurrence it was now more copious and went on longer or at least long enough for his wife (he had married Eileen O'Shaughnessy in 1936) to think something should be done, even if Orwell didn't. He avoided doctors and hospitals and was unforthcoming about his medical history when examined. His brother-in-law, Laurence O'Shaughnessy, was instrumental in Orwell's admission to Preston Hall, a British Legion-run sanatorium, at Maidstone, Kent where he was a consultant thoracic surgeon. Orwell was examined and X-rayed, and his sputum cultured. The eventual diagnosis of tuberculosis surprised him: 'I have an old lesion in one lung [left] which has been there at any rate 10 years & was never discovered before because I am non-infectious, i.e. no bacteria to show.' He remained optimistic: 'I don't think there's really much wrong with me.' He was 35 years old.

Tuberculosis is spread by the expelled secretions from the lungs or larynx (voice-box) of the patient. Coughs, sneezes, and even speech create aerosols of tiny airborne particles. These evaporate to 'droplet nuclei' of less than 1 micrometre in size, which contain the tubercle bacilli and are inhaled. The minimum time one must spend with a single active tuberculosis patient—the index case—before acquiring the disease is unknown, but evidence suggests that it can be brief. Nor do we know the duration of exposure after which it is inevitable that infection will take place. Some people have become infected on flights lasting more than eight hours.[3] One recent study based

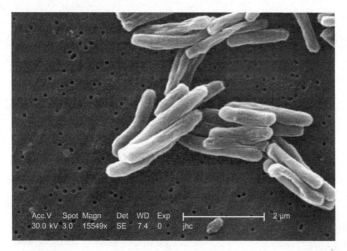

1. Magnified nearly 16,000 times, the rod-shaped *Mycobacterium tuberculosis* as seen with a scanning electron microscope: to think that something so small could cause so much suffering. (CDC/ Dr Ray Butler)

on an outbreak in a school, the Crown Hills Community College in Leicester, indicated that in this case spending 130 hours of shared room air with an index case resulted in transmission. Crowded rooms with more than one tuberculous case obviously increase the risks and this 130-hour period need not be uninterrupted.[4]

Carried along with the inspired air, the bacteria travel down into the lungs, coming to rest in the furthest reaches of the lungs, the tiny air sacs or alveoli. Their presence here stimulates the immune system. The macrophages (specialized cells of the immune system) ingest the *M. tuberculosis* but don't kill them. The bacilli multiply within these cells, although they are slow-growing, dividing every twenty to twenty-four hours (bacterial division rates are usually measured in minutes). These cells eventually split open, releasing an increased number of bacteria, which are again engulfed. This process usually lasts for a period of weeks during which the bacilli can spread elsewhere in the lungs, to the lymph nodes nearest the lungs and to other parts of the body. This general immune activity (macrophages ingest all foreign material entering the lungs) is followed after a few weeks by a more specific response, which can result in the intracellular killing of the bacilli. This killing takes place within a walled-off granuloma or nodule (a chronic inflammatory lesion made up essentially of immune system cells). In most infected people (90–95 per cent) tuberculosis is now contained. These latent cases show no clinical or laboratory signs of disease, are not infectious because there are no bacilli in their sputum, and may never suffer again from their infection. In the minority of cases (5–10 per cent) the disease is not contained. The slow proliferation of the bacilli in the body continues, probably reaching a symptomatic level in two years or less. This is known as primary tuberculosis. Of the initially luckier infected majority, over time the disease will flare up in about 5 per cent of cases—reactivation tuberculosis. It is also possible to acquire a second infection from an external source.

Those most at risk have always been the underprivileged—often malnourished and subject to poor working and living conditions, where overcrowding is common. Smokers, alcoholics, and injecting drug users are in greater danger, as are those who suffer from diabetes, end-stage kidney disease, another lung disease such as silicosis or who have a depressed immune system most commonly today as a result of medication or HIV infection. Age is important too. Children with primary tuberculosis tend to develop more severe disease, which is often dispersed throughout the body and includes a greater incidence of meningeal tuberculosis in the membranes surrounding the brain. As heavy milk drinkers, infants and children are traditionally more exposed to the bovine strain of tuberculosis, *Mycobacterium bovis*, which is found in unpasteurized milk from infected cattle. Hence the current concern in the UK with badgers transmitting tuberculosis to cows. Children also pick up tuberculosis in the same way as adults, through the respiratory tract. In women the demands of menstruation and child-bearing increase the toll of tuberculosis.

In the early years of the 20th century the mortality and morbidity from tuberculosis in Britain were declining. The great killer of industrialization and rapid urbanization was on the wane. The fall was not the same across the social classes—the poor suffered and died more than the rich. Someone from Orwell's comfortable enough middle-class background—father in the Indian Civil Service; mother the daughter of a merchant in Burma; able to afford good food and medical care when needed—might have stood less chance of infection. There was a tuberculous aunt, but she died before he was born. It was still easy enough for the young Orwell to have picked up his tuberculosis from his Indian nanny or the wider community or at boarding school.

His opportunities for acquiring tuberculosis and/or reactivating an old lesion substantially increased as an adult. Orwell blamed the Burmese climate for 'ruining his health' without specifying why. Today Myanmar (Burma) has a high burden of tuberculosis, but estimates for the 1920s are unreliable. The prison population, with which his job brought him into contact, would probably have had a higher incidence of tuberculosis as a result of crowding, poor hygiene, and meagre food. Outdoors, on tour, should have been healthier from a tuberculosis perspective. Back in temperate Europe, as part of his life as a would-be writer he 'sometimes lived for months on end amongst the poor and half criminal elements who inhabit the worst parts of the poorer quarters or take to the streets, begging and stealing'.[5] Even off the streets he endured 'several years of fairly severe poverty'.[6] Orwell was generally free of much of the co-morbidity associated with tuberculosis. He lived in the era before HIV, which is such a significant problem today. His chronic bronchitis, later diagnosed as bronchiectasis, was likely to be significant. Bronchiectasis involves dilation of the bronchial tubes in the lungs, resulting in a reduced ability to remove secretions upwards. These then pool in the lower regions of the lungs and make an ideal environment for bacterial infections to proliferate. His living conditions, nutritional status, addiction to smoking his own cigarettes 'rolled from the strongest, coarsest black shag pipe tobacco' (a considerable irritant to lungs struggling to remove secretions) together presented plenty of high-risk opportunities to contract tuberculosis or to reactivate an old lesion and turn latent tuberculosis into active disease.[7] It is quite likely that this had happened when Orwell was hospitalized on 18 March 1938.

He had to reconstruct his medical history for the examining doctors at Preston Hall—the lack of contact with a regular practitioner as a result of his somewhat erratic lifestyle and a less structured approach to medical care at this time made his records patchy. The discussion of a ten-year-old lesion is a better indication of chronicity rather than a precise indication of the time of infection. But he was clearly in acutely poor health. In addition to coughing up blood, at six foot three inches tall (1.9 m), he weighed only 159 lb (72.12 kg). Even though confirmation from the laboratory was delayed and then inconclusive (*M. tuberculosis* is a slow and fastidious grower *in vitro*), Orwell was immediately treated as a tuberculosis patient. He expected to be at Preston Hall for three months, but stayed for over five. Initially ordered complete bedrest with no writing, he spent his time doing crosswords and 'studying botany in a very elementary way'.[8] At the beginning of September 1938, on medical advice, Orwell left for Morocco to overwinter in a warm climate. From his villa outside Marrakech he reported feeling better and started writing again (*Coming Up for Air*). But he was ill in January 1939 after a week's trip to the Atlas Mountains and again in April immediately after returning to England. These short periods of ill health continued but it appeared that his body had once again contained the active tuberculosis, or he was at least able was able to plough on anyway. He had been prescribed 'M & B', probably sulfapyridine, a sulpha drug active against other bacteria (but not the *M. tuberculosis*) infecting his lungs and adding to his general pulmonary troubles.

When war broke out Orwell volunteered for the army, but was rejected because of his lungs. He believed his involvement in the Spanish Civil War kept him from a desk job in the services. Bitterly disappointed not to be able to contribute directly to the war effort, he joined the Home Guard (May 1940) and the Indian Section of the BBC's Eastern Service (August 1941). He resigned from both in November 1943, from the Home Guard on grounds of health. Almost immediately he took over the literary editorship of the left-wing weekly *Tribune* and began to write *Animal Farm*—the book that would transform his literary career. Life became more complicated in May 1944 when the Orwells adopted the month-old Richard Horatio Blair. Less than a year later (March 1945) Eileen died under anaesthesia during an operation. Orwell was in a Paris hospital when he learned the tragic news: he had gone to Europe as a war correspondent.

Throughout the war his chronic ill health had continued. He had lost his regular thoracic specialist when his brother-in-law was killed during the evacuation of Dunkirk in June 1940. Living with sickness for so long, he may have been the last to notice its cumulative effects, although he promised to finish the *Animal Farm* manuscript on time 'unless I get ill or something'.[9] In 1944, after walking for 500 yards at a 'rather fast pace', his chest could be heard 'whistling' for five minutes as he sat and recovered.[10] A telling comment from a friend revealed that for a man supposedly so obsessed about smell (it is a frequent trope of his sensory descriptions) and middle-class prejudices about the assumed smell of the lower orders, it was Orwell who stank: 'It was the rotting lungs that you could smell, not at once, but increasingly as the evening wore on, in a confined room; a sweetish smell of decay.'[11] In February 1946, after a winter of hard work in the wake of *Animal Farm*'s success, Orwell's housekeeper found him walking down the corridor of his flat in Islington with blood coming from his mouth. He was haemorrhaging (bleeding) in his lungs again. Susan Watson fetched a jug of ice-water, wrapped a block of ice in a cloth, which he placed on his forehead, and sat holding his hand until the bleeding stopped.

Haemoptysis—coughing up the haemorrhaged blood—is one of the signs of active pulmonary tuberculosis. Orwell's bronchiectasis and tendency to develop pneumonia could also cause blood to appear in the sputum, but the tuberculosis was at work here. The lungs bleed because, over time, the repeated breakdown of granulomas, releasing *M. tuberculosis* bacilli, pus, and dead tissues creates increasingly large and numerous cavities in the lung tissue. It is an unceasing battle of attrition between body cells and bacilli in part mediated by the nature of the immune response. The cavities may become the sites of further infection (tuberculous or another bacteria/virus) or eat into blood vessels or airways. The more extensive the destruction caused by this cavitation process, the greater the duration and intensity of the bleeding. The more debilitated the patient already is, the harder it is to recover. Each destructive bout reduces the amount of functional lung tissue and hence the body's ability to oxygenate itself. In between bouts scar tissue of a fibrotic or calcified nature may reform and 'harden' the lungs.

The other most frequently experienced symptoms are a cough producing sputum, fever (commonly 'low-grade' or a slight rise in temperature), night-sweats, malaise, weight loss with wasting (cachexia) even when the appetite is not diminished, and difficult or laboured breathing (dyspnoea). A hacking cough exhausts and causes soreness in the ribs. Chest pain is not always a prominent feature, but infected pleura (the membranes surrounding the lungs) do hurt a lot.

After this haemorrhage episode Orwell reluctantly took to his bed for two weeks, but avoided telling the attending doctor—who diagnosed 'gastritis'—his tubercular history. He was planning his return in May with family and furniture to Barnhill, the cottage he had rented for a holiday in September 1945, and did not want to be institutionalized in a sanatorium. Barnhill on the isle of Jura, in the Scottish Inner Hebrides, was remote with rather primitive amenities, but Orwell loved the isolation and freedom from the continual pressure of his increasingly successful literary life. The plan for Jura was to 'do no work or writing or anything of the kind for two months. I feel desperately tired and jaded.'[12] In October Orwell returned to London to pick up his old routine, for what would be one of the coldest winters on record.

He had begun to write 1984 at the end of the Jura summer in 1946 and left again for the island in April 1947. This time he flew across Scotland. The world was moving on. In and out of bed, he continued to work in a haze of cigarette smoke. Visibly becoming frailer, he continued to watch his son grow, although he was advised not to let the boy come too close to him, so as to prevent passing on the germs. At least no one suggested the boy should be taken away from him completely. He worked in the garden if possible—permanent help was now on hand in the shape of his future brother-in-law Bill Dunn—and persisted with the manuscript. Progress was slower than he wanted in May: 'I have not got as far as I hoped…because I have really been in most wretched health this year since about January (my chest as usual) and can't quite shake it off.' It was much the same in September: 'I've been in wretched health…my chest as usual—starting with last winter.'[13] Orwell finished the novel's first draft in October and, near collapse, called in a chest specialist in November—'I dare not make the journey to the mainland while I have a temperature.' He accepted his doctor's advice and admitted himself as soon as possible to a sanatorium—Hairmyres Hospital, East Kilbride near Glasgow—in December. It was a time of reckoning and realization.

Orwell finally acknowledged that he had serious tuberculosis. He had a large cavity in the left lung and a smaller area at the top of the right. As he was infectious, Richard was to be kept away. Learning about the risks of unpasteurized milk, he sought a tuberculin-tested cow for Barnhill. That was the easy bit. Orwell's treatment moved beyond the rest cure of 1938, although he was confined to bed with no typewriter. Bruce Dick ordered a phrenic nerve crush disabling the diaphragm on the side of the diseased lung. The collapsed lung was supposed to rest and hopefully to heal. The desired position of the diaphragm was achieved and maintained by air injected into the pleural cavity. Artificial pneumothorax had been an increasingly popular interventionist therapy since the 1930s partly because it often reduced sputum production and hence infectivity. It was also painful and debilitating. But the night-sweats ameliorated and he began to regain some of the approximately 28 lb (12.7 kg) he had lost. There was a further rationale for resting the lung— getting into as good a shape as possible to try a new therapy— the antibiotic drug streptomycin. It had been marketed in the USA in 1946, but Britain was too poor to buy adequate supplies for its tuberculous population. Through his friendship with David Astor, editor/owner of the *Observer* newspaper, Orwell secured a supply, which he bought with the American proceeds of *Animal Farm* lodged in a dollar account in the USA. It was close but no cigar. Although there was apparent improvement, the streptomycin was discontinued when Orwell suffered an allergic reaction. This drug, which in a combination therapy would render tuberculosis essentially a curable disease, part of the postwar miracle of modern medicine, was not for him. The medical staff at Hairmyres gradually got him out of bed, out of doors, and then out of hospital. In July 1948 he returned to Barnhill and the typewriter.

Orwell finished a final typed copy of 1984 at the end of the year, and promptly took to his bed full time—he reported in October already spending half the day there. He would not really get up again. He wrote to Warburg (his publisher) in his charac-teristic understated tone, 'I am really very unwell indeed.'[14]

Throughout the dismal summer his activities were increasingly circumscribed by ill health: 'To walk even a few hundred yards promptly upsets me … I cannot so much as pull up a weed in the garden … I can't type much because it tires me too much to sit up at table.' A typical tubercular decline with touches of an author's special problems. The fever was back and he was losing weight. After Christmas at home, he left Jura in the first days of 1949 for the Cranham Lodge Sanatorium in the Cotswolds, Gloucestershire. Here in a private chalet—he was now able to pay reasonably well for his care and wanted the privacy to work, although again the typewriter was forbidden—the doctors unsuccessfully tried the next new anti-tuberculous drug, PAS (para-aminosalicylic acid). There was no scope for further surgical intervention—both of his lungs were now too compromised.

To his disgust and dismay the frequency of the haemorrhages increased and the doctors tried streptomycin again. The allergic reaction was swifter and severer than before. It was discontinued. While Orwell valiantly ran his life (with help) from his sanatorium bed, 'too feverish to go over to the X-ray room & stand up against the screen', he continued to plan his next novel and think about the future: 'The only thing that worries me about my financial position is the possibility that I might become like some of the people here, i.e. able to stay alive but unable to work.'[15] He remained optimistic, convinced that he could and sometimes did improve. His solution was to move in September to the private wing of one the country's leading hospitals, University College Hospital, Gower Street, London and to get married again: 'I suppose everyone will be horrified, but apart from other considerations I really think I should stay alive longer if I were married.'[16]

Sonia Brownell was the last of a series of women the lonely Orwell had proposed to in the years after Eileen's death. They were married on 13 October 1949. Orwell practically pointed out that it would be easier to travel with her as his wife when he went abroad to Switzerland the next year. Despite the encouraging comments of his doctors (who privately gave him little chance), Orwell didn't live to use the new fishing rod standing ready in the corner of his room. After a massive final pulmonary haemorrhage leading to shock and asphyxia, he died alone in his hospital bed.

Orwell's final haemorrhage spared him the possible further dissemination of the disease in other parts of his body. Carried by the bloodstream or lymphatic system, either during the initial infection with M. *tuberculosis* or as a result of reactivation, the bacilli can progress as in the lungs to form containing granulomas or active cavities. Extrapulmonary tuberculosis occurs in about 15 to 20 per cent of adult cases where the immune system is not compromised. In the immuno-suppressed (and children) the tendency to spread is much greater. Beyond the lungs and the membranes that surround them, the most common forms of extrapulmonary tuberculosis are found in the lymphatic system, especially the glands of the neck (cervical or supraclavicular chains) where the resulting swellings and disfigurement are known as scrofula. Other visible manifestations are found in the bones and joints. Pott's disease, with its classic curvature of the spine, is caused by the destruction of the vertebrae, frequently in the thoracic part of the spine. Marcel 'Max' Blecher's spinal tuberculosis was diagnosed at the age of 19 in 1928. The solution was to encase him in a plaster cast. This artificial exoskeleton pinned him to his bed as surely as if had been an upturned beetle. Getting out involved being transferred to an elaborate horse-drawn cart. He died in 1938. Tuberculosis of the genito-urinary tract involves the now familiar processes of cavitation, tissue necrosis, and bleeding. The same thing happens in the gastrointestinal tract, to which it often spreads when patients swallow their own bacilli-laden sputum. Everywhere it is ultimately painful, unpleasant, degrading, and deadly.

Orwell died on the cusp of a new, more positive era in the history of tuberculosis. Improvements in the standard of living coupled with the anti-tuberculosis drugs (despite proving so disappointing for him) transformed the experience of tuberculosis in the developed world. Orwell gave his unused streptomycin to two other patients who recovered. Able to act against foci of bacilli anywhere in the body, and providing the tissue damage was not too extensive, patients began to recover when previously they had died. With viable drugs in the dispensary and programmes for early case detection the downward trend of tuberculosis accelerated. Fewer active cases further reduced the rate of new infections. The sanatoria emptied. Tuberculosis became a thing of the past for most of the population in the developed world, but even here it did not go away and as ever the developing world fared much worse.

It came as a surprise when tuberculosis and its new forms, multi-drug-resistant (MDRTB) and extensively drug-resistant (XDRTB) tuberculosis, were included among the newly re-emergent diseases of the late 20th and 21st centuries. It should not have done. After all it is an ancient global disease, apparently controllable, in specific circumstances, for a mere four or five decades, with massive effort. In 2010 there were between '8.5–9.2 million cases and 1.2–1.5 million deaths' from tuberculosis. With 3 billion (a third of the world's population) exposed to the bacteria, a huge pool of latent infection exists.[17]

I

ANCIENT BACTERIA, OLD DISEASES

There's Always Been a Lot of Mycobacteria Out There

Some 300 million years ago it seems that the common ancestor of today's species of mycobacteria began to live in close association with a range of animals. These parasitic forms became dependent on their hosts for survival. As is the nature of parasitism, they exacted a toll on the host: disease and/or premature death. Other species retained the ancestral habit, remaining at large in the environment in fresh water, soil, dust, and peat bogs. The majority lived (and live today) as saprophytes—on dead and decaying matter—indeed some environmental mycobacteria may well prove to be important in the future manufacture of biofuels.

Among the parasites, most important for the history of human disease are *Mycobacterium leprae* and the *Mycobacterium tuberculosis* complex (MBTC). *M. leprae* causes leprosy. The *Mycobacterium tuberculosis* complex includes *M. tuberculosis*, *M. africanum*, *M. bovis*, and *M. canettii*. All can cause tuberculosis. Each member of the MBTC has a preferred mammalian host and a slightly different appearance (the phenotype). They appear to be an extremely consistent bunch at the genetic level (the genotype), which usually means they are the clonal descendants of a single successful ancestor. The date for their emergence is currently set at 20,000–35,000 years ago. What was happening before this is actively being explored.[1]

The bit players are the non-tuberculosis mycobacteria (NTM), a term used for all the other disease-causing but free-living species. These can produce an extensive range of ailments including inflammation of the lymph node (lymphadenitis), skin diseases, tuberculosis-like pulmonary disease, inflammation of the bones (osteomyelitis), and post-traumatic wound infections. Besides direct illness, historical exposure to these related bacteria might have affected the evolution of the immune response to the tuberculosis-causing bacilli. Non-tuberculosis mycobacteria also cause post-operative infections linked to catheter use and the diverse infections and disseminated diseases in the immuno-compromised. These pathologies reflect new human associations with ancient organisms, the side effects of modern invasive medicine, and the changing nature of the human disease profile—most spectacularly the rise of the HIV/AIDS epidemic in the last thirty years.

It is argued that as today's vertebrates evolved those harbouring the early mycobacteria carried them along, host and parasite developing together—vertical transmission. It used to be confidently and quite reasonably thought that M. *tuberculosis* mutated from the closely allied M. *bovis* of cattle and goats, spreading to humans by a horizontal transfer when we began domesticating these animals about 9000 BCE in the Neolithic. This is a familiar model in the history of infectious diseases: a zoonosis (one initially spread from animals to people) becomes a permanent part of the human disease economy. The specificity of M. *tuberculosis* for humans rather than the more omnipresent M. *bovis* was interpreted as supporting evidence.

Larger groups of humans generally lived more settled lifestyles as members of herding communities. They potentially enjoyed more regular sources of protein from the meat and especially the milk of the ruminants. On the downside, giving up the mobile small-group hunter-gatherer lifestyle brought a greater proximity to other people and to M. *bovis*. In cattle M. *bovis* bacteria caused (and causes) a chronic disease although the animal remained useful. Ingested by humans in milk or meat, this organism produced what we would recognize as tuberculosis, with the gut and the nearby lymph nodes as the primary sites of infection. Cows also cough and out of this germ pool, it was postulated, mutations of M. *bovis* became adapted, as M. *tuberculosis*, to the oxygen-rich environment of the human lung. Once lodged here, the bacteria became capable of spreading directly between one human and the next and, in effect, a new form of disease predominantly targeting the pulmonary system came into being.

So far so good, but recent DNA sequencing of the M. *tuberculosis* genome suggests a rather different evolutionary path for the *Mycobacterium tuberculosis* complex and therefore the human disease's history. Some of the older model still pertains—M. *bovis* was (and remains) a source of infection; population density plays a significant role in the transmission of pulmonary tuberculosis. But it is now suggested that a human germ has been around rather longer than its cattle equivalent. Instead of M. *tuberculosis* being a mutation of M. *bovis*, analysis of the genomes suggests that M. *tuberculosis* is the older of the two, M. *bovis* evolving via the ancestor of M. *africanum*, one of the other human tuberculosis-causing species.[2] This ancestral bacterial organism may well have been bothering our hominin precursors in East Africa with tuberculosis-like illness. Thus a hominin-derived rather than animal-derived pathogen could be responsible for much of our modern experience of tuberculosis. As well as potentially explaining the past, this has implications for assisting with current epidemiological puzzles, such as the effective geographical range of the BCG vaccination.[3]

Whatever their origin, all mycobacteria have evolved a unique thick cell wall made from glycolipids and lipids. These waxy molecules are part of the group's evolutionary success rendering them safe from assault. They help the bacteria resist long exposure to acids and alkalis; guard against splitting or lysis by proteins in body fluids; and protect against antibiotics like penicillin, which do battle by destroying the cell coat of many other common disease-causing bacteria. In the bacterial pantheon, mycobacteria are slow growers. *Escherichia coli* takes only twenty minutes to divide itself into two, a further twenty minutes for these two to become four, and so on. *M. tuberculosis* requires twenty to twenty-four hours to divide once. It routinely takes over seven days for a colony to become clearly visible to the naked eye.

Such sluggard division is the result of the cell wall's complexity. When preparing to divide, the many layers of the cell wall must be synthesized, but the rod-like shape maintained. Then careful management of the breakdown of the existing cell wall components to maintain integrity throughout division is necessary, all the while responding to unfavourable changes in the surrounding environment. The slowness of cell division and its fine control are part of the chronic nature of tuberculosis. So too are the persistent but often subclinical infection and the trick of dormancy with the ability to break this stasis when opportune. All these strategies appear to be modulated by sensitive feedback loops. Lipid-rich cell walls have a further utility in the history of tuberculosis—it is likely that this feature makes the bacteria extremely resistant to degradation over very long periods of time. With due care their ancient DNA (aDNA) can be extracted, amplified, and used as proof of the presence of disease in the appropriate context in humans and animals.

The key words for mycobacteria are longevity, resilience, and ubiquity. Welcome to the world of tuberculosis.

A Prehistoric Scourge

Knowledge of the long history of human interactions with mycobacteria comes from a variety of sources. These have been interwoven into histories of disease, human settlement, social development, war, and conquest. Under due scrutiny bones and mummies can provide evidence of what we understand as historical tuberculosis. Some are more unequivocal than others. There has been and remains an understandable temptation to fit the facts to convenient 'just so stories' which locate the history of tuberculosis into a wider historical narrative. So bearing this in mind, over to the bones, bodies, and ancient DNA.

Mycobacteria leave certain marks on bones and soft tissues. Visual inspections by palaeosteologists (bioarchaeologists in the USA) who study ancient bones and palaeopathologists had the bacteria present and interacting deleteriously with their human hosts from at least around 5800 BCE. This is the age (plus or minus 90 years) of the oldest tuberculous skeletal remains among a collection from Liguria, Italy.[4] Often the spine provided proof for infection most dramatically when the degenerated and fused thoracic (occasionally lumbar) vertebrae collapsed into a sharp angular deformity (kyphosis) and gave its victim a hunchback during life. The unfortunate but now famous Nesperehan, an Egyptian priest of the Twenty-first Dynasty (1100 BCE), had a pronounced hunchback and a psoas abscess. This pus-filled swelling attached to the psoas muscle of the back is highly characteristic of a modern diagnosis of extrapulmonary tuberculosis. Lesions on the ribs—on the internal surface, where the membrane surrounding the bone has become inflamed following contact with tuberculous lung tissue—can be read as markers of the pulmonary form.[5] Less frequently but very usefully, as in the case of an ancient Nubian woman from the island of Hesa, preserved soft tissues—a collapsed lung and fibrous adhesions—alert historians to the presence of what we think of as the most common pulmonary type of tuberculosis.

Around the world burial sites and preserved bodies hinted at how widespread tuberculosis may have been. In the Old World, material from Poland, Spain, Russia, Greece, Thailand, China, and Denmark followed Italy and Egypt on the tubercular map, as the Neolithic became the Bronze and then the Iron Age. The pattern of spread seemed to follow the developing civilization and urbanization, which stretched out from the Fertile Crescent in the Near East. One by one most of the other countries of Europe and Asia can be added through the centuries of the first millennium CE to the later medieval period. By this time tuberculosis appears to have become endemic, an ever-present smouldering cause of sickness and death. Its effects were masked to some extent by the ravages of the acute infectious diseases. However, what we might be sampling is the development of burial practices over time and place as much as the spread of the disease.

In the New World tuberculosis left its calling cards too. The increasing numbers of tuberculous mummies apparently dating from the first millennium CE, conserved by hot, dry conditions in Peru and Chile, proved to be something of a conundrum. Tuberculosis, it used to be thought, had not entered continental America in the first wave of human occupation towards the end of the last glacial period perhaps 17,000–10,000 years ago. It was assumed that active cases would be lost in the natural wastage on the initial stages of the journey from the Old to New World and any latent cases would then have succumbed to the 'cold screen' endured by the survivors as they crossed the Bering Land Bridge. It was posited instead that tuberculosis came as part of the Columbian Exchange of the late 15th and early 16th centuries when the Spanish and Portuguese accidentally discovered and conquered South America on their way to India. The invaders wreaked havoc with the germs they carried— smallpox, measles, and tuberculosis—among the immunologically naïve locals and took syphilis home with them in return, hence the 'exchange'.

Preliminary investigations looked merely for the presence of acid-fast bacilli. Acid-fastness refers to a characteristic of some bacteria, when dyed, to increase their visibility under the microscope and crucially includes the mycobacteria. Where acid-fast bacilli were found in the context of the appropriate lesions— tell-tale pathological damage—they gave reasonable evidence for the presence of mycobacteria and hence tuberculosis. The recovery of such organisms in 1973 from a mummy in Southern Peru with a reliable radiocarbon date of 700 CE promoted a (somewhat reluctant) reassessment of the history of tuberculosis in South America. Subsequent developments in aDNA recovery and polymerase chain reaction (PCR) amplification substantiated the challenge: M. tuberculosis complex bacteria in South America had caused tuberculosis-like illnesses from at least 2000 BCE in Chile.[6] How did the disease originate if it had not been brought by the conquistadors? Did it come with earlier landings on the Pacific coast from Asia and Oceania? More needs to be done here as the history of the peopling of the Americas is revised, but the longevity of the disease is now beyond doubt.

What of North America, where the Native American's similar decimation by 'imported' infectious diseases led to the assumption that they too had no prior exposure to tuberculosis? The skeletal evidence from large settlements at Norris Farms in the Illinois River Valley dated to 1300 CE, for instance, has been sufficient to allow estimates of tuberculosis's endemicity in a specific population. A supplementary PCR technique—spoligotyping—confirming both the presence and the strain of the Mycobacterium tuberculosis complex is providing material for partial answers and it seems that the bovines might be partly to blame after all. Not for passing on M. bovis though. Spoligotyping of aDNA from a long-dead (17,000 years BP) American bison with characteristic tubercular lesions reveals the likelihood that this animal was infected with the precursor of the Mycobacterium tuberculosis complex. Further sampling of other animals from the same source in Wyoming—bighorn sheep and musk ox—indicates that the animals that wandered over the Bering Strait during the Pleistocene carried the pathogen with them and that it was widespread.[7]

Back in the Old World during the past twenty years many of the previously scrutinized bones and bodies have been reinvestigated using the developing aDNA techniques. As a result some would like to move the earliest case back to 9,000 years ago from a Neolithic settlement in Atlit-Yam in the Eastern Mediterranean—a submerged village off the coast of present-day Israel. Here the bones of a mother and child who both died of tuberculosis (determined by the bone lesions and presence of aDNA) were found along with those of extensive animal remains. Here the shift to fishing, farming, and animal keeping apparently supported a population density capable of maintaining a settled village life and endemic as opposed to sporadic tuberculosis.[8]

If prehistoric tuberculosis seems old, there is an interesting debate about some tuberculosis-like lesions on a fossilised *Homo erectus* skull. Found near Kocabaş, Turkey, it is *c.*500,000 years old. The difficulty of being sure the lesions result from tubercular meningitis, without other supporting evidence, reminds us how hard it is to confidently reconstruct the deep history of disease. If this appears to be too early for the presence of modern M. *tuberculosis* (thought to be *c.*35,000 years old), the ancestral progenitor species from which it developed its cunning complexities, is estimated to be perhaps three million years old: plenty of time to dog the proto-human race.

New ways of investigating the history of M. *tuberculosis* enhance knowledge about the germ's past. Serendipitous finds of ancient material can drive back the tuberculosis timeline, reconfiguring aspects of the disease's record. We continue to unpack and then repack a construction of the history of tuberculosis, but it quickly becomes a history of the mycobacteria rather than the experience of disease. Tantalizing as the prehistoric period may be for modern bacteriology, we need to return closer to the present, to the early written records to more fully appreciate the disease in its human terms. Modern bacteriological reinterpretations may provide greater certainty in retrospective diagnosis

9

but they cannot rewrite the recorded experiences of those who coughed, sweated, and bled from their lungs, suffered disintegrating bones and joints, and shrinking of the flesh. These people explained and experienced such phenomena in different, non-bacteriological ways, which made sense to them. It is time to give up the specificity of the mycobacteria for a while and begin to speak the language of phthisis, consumption, and the humours.

Phthisis: All-Consuming Consumption in the Ancient World

The understanding of disease in the ancient world was fundamentally different from ours, varying both over time and among the diverse cultures of Asia and the Mediterranean basin. The belief that disease was divinely inspired and treatable through supplication of the gods was a shared characteristic. Beginning in the classical period in the 5th century BCE such celestial explanations were challenged by a new naturalism. Temple cults of healing continued, but various groups devised secular explanations for health and disease. The physicians who collected around Hippocrates of Cos (c.460–c.370 BCE) introduced humoral medicine. Based on a theoretical configuration of body fluids, it was rooted in the dominant philosophy of matter. Everything in the sublunary world, including the human body, was made up of the four elements—fire, water, air, and earth. In a healthy body the humours were in a state of balance, but during illness this was upset and the goal of treatment was to restore it where possible. Humoral medicine gained the ascendency over its competitors and lasted a very long time—effectively until the 18th century in the western medical tradition—largely thanks to its greatest exponent and most efficient codifier, Galen of Pergamon (129–c.210 CE).

From the sometimes contradictory Hippocratic writings (not all written by Hippocrates himself) Galen distilled a wonderfully neat scheme of four humours—blood, yellow bile, black bile, and phlegm, which he linked with the four elements and the four qualities—hot, dry, cold, and wet. There was also a time component. The humours followed the seasons of each year and people passed through the same sequence during their lifetime. Thus spring and childhood were dominated by hot, wet blood: winter and old age by cold, wet phlegm. The mutability of illnesses, an important part of humoral pathology, could be explained in part by these progressions.

An individual had an exclusive humoral blueprint and his or her experience of ill health was correspondingly unique. There were diseased individuals rather than diseases, but since there could be only so much variation along the assorted continua of humoral medicine's framework, distinctive patterns could be distilled by observant doctors into pen-portraits of disease. What we know about the disease experience in this period is essentially dominated by these texts, which articulated the likely cause, course, and outcome of the illnesses the Greeks recognized.

There was also advice on treatment. Determinedly holistic, humoral therapy was concerned with rebalancing the humours and regulating the six non-naturals: air (surrounding atmosphere), diet, exercise, sleep, wastes (excretions), and emotions. Preventive medicine aimed to maintain an individual's ideal humoral balance within the body and its relation to the world via the non-naturals. Rebalancing of the humours called for the application of opposites: allopathy. Cooling remedies might be advised for a fever, the result of an excess of the hot, wet humour—blood. Reduction of the fire in the body, by removal of the humoral excess—letting blood—could be employed. A natural bloodletting—haemorrhage—was therefore not always considered a bad sign. Such active intervention was tempered by the Greeks' belief in the healing power of nature: sometimes it was better to do nothing but care for or nurse the patient. Accurate prognoses, a significant feature of these texts, helped doctors manage their cases and prepared patients for what they could expect.

Appropriately sifted, there is sufficient evidence in the Greek canon for the familiar Orwellian symptoms of coughing, haemoptysis, fever, and weight loss and for much of the range of non-pulmonary symptoms that he was spared including the dissipated miliary form of the disease (comparable material has also been extricated from the Chinese, Ayurvedic, Babylonian, and Assyrian texts). It is therefore possible to extrapolate backwards and apply modern knowledge to ancient texts, constructing with some certainty retrospective diagnoses of, say, pulmonary tuberculosis (perhaps with gastric sequelae); Pott's disease of the spine; tubercular lymphadenitis, or scrofula. All the while we are aware that these are members of the tuberculosis family, each caused by the same infectious agent working on different parts of the body: different manifestations of the same disease. This has no meaning for the Greeks. So what did wasting and haemorrhaging from the lungs, a deformed spine, and chronic, perhaps suppurating, masses in the neck mean some two millennia ago?

We know from the Hippocratic corpus that the Greeks suffered from phthisis. By the time these texts were composed, phthisis was sufficiently widespread to be included in the

Epidemics. The title referred less to those explosions of infectious disease we know as 'epidemics' than to those that were commonly present everywhere—ubiquitous, established diseases. Such an entrenched position meshes with what we know from etymology. The word that became *phthinein* as the ancient Greek language developed during the second millennium BCE, had arrived in the Balkan Peninsula with the Indo-European invaders, towards the end of the third millennium BCE. A general word for waning, in its medical garb it came to mean a chronic wasting away (especially the muscles), atrophying, being consumed, declining, rotting. All described what happened to the body of the phthisic (a person suffering from phthisis).

An emphasis on slow bodily consumption—as in the melting away of the flesh or using up of the body—was not restricted to medical texts. In Homer's *Odyssey*—the epic telling of the hero's return from Troy—the poet referred to a 'grievous consumption', which took the soul from the body; and to one who 'lies in sickness...a long time wasting away'.[10] Aristophanes (4th century BCE), among others, used 'consumptive' as a term of abuse in his play *The Assemblywomen*. Wasting diseases, atrophy of the bones and flesh were afflictions the Israelites faced, as recorded in the Old Testament books of Leviticus and Deuteronomy. Again etymology is helpful: *schachepheth*—the ancient Hebrew word for a wasting disease; its derivative—*schachefet*—the contemporary Hebrew term for tuberculosis.

It is reasonable to suppose that such references to wasting included Greek phthisis, which in turn may have included modern pulmonary tuberculosis. However, they also incorporated a disparate range of conditions that exhausted and drained the body of its life and flesh. Illnesses that heightened the body's metabolic demands and/or suppressed the appetite, especially over a prolonged period—anaemias, cancers, diabetes, low-grade infections—may have been covered by this umbrella term. Consumption could also refer to the dissolution of specific parts of the body: spines, hips, larynxes, and kidneys. If consumption thus compels a breadth of meaning, phthisis itself was not a single disease. Medical authors in the classical period listed the various types of phthisis they recognized, their origins, and how they were differentiated from other diseases. The overlap with pulmonary tuberculosis is extensive but not exhaustive, as samples from the Hippocratic corpus illustrate.

Book I of *Diseases* recorded three kinds of phthisis. The first was linked to a previous empyema—a collection of pus in a body cavity, especially the pleural cavity surrounding the lungs—and an excess of the cold, wet, watery humour phlegm. Patients who suffered an inflammation of the lungs, and could not rid themselves of superfluous sputum and phlegm, developed an ulceration there. Choking and difficulty in breathing, typically using only the upper part of the chest, followed. Eventually the overabundant phlegm closed the respiratory passage and death ensued. An empyema might also occur when excess phlegm fell from the brain (the organ identified with this humour) to the lungs. While the patient noticed a slight cough, somewhat bitter sputum, and an occasional, moderate fever, the lungs became increasingly irritated and ulcerated as the phlegm adhered to the tissues, and purulence set in. Heaviness of the chest, sometimes pain (perhaps extreme to the front and back of the thorax), and a heating of the body came next. A raised temperature attracted the phlegm from the rest of the body in a bid to cool the lungs. In health, the lungs served to cool the blood with which the inspired air was mixed; in phthisis this function was impaired. With perceptibly thicker and more putrid matter in the lungs, phthisics expelled this as best they could by coughing or 'vomiting' it up, but the body was now in a dreadful loop. The more purulent and copious the matter, the higher the temperature rose and the greater the frequency and violence of the cough. Patients lacked appetite and the wasting of the flesh was stark, but so long as they could continue to expel the putrid matter there was hope. If phlegm's downward tendency spread to the bowels, digestion of what little food could be taken was disordered and death followed.

The second kind of phthisis came on after a burst blood vessel. The blood, transformed into purulent matter, caused ulceration in the lungs and a similar course unfolded. Herodotus, the 5th-century BCE historian, perhaps described such a case when he told of the demise of Pharnunches, riding out in haste from Sardis to meet his command under the Persians. Thrown from his horse, he began to spit up blood and 'the disease turned into consumption'.[11] The third kind resulted from an acute inflammation of the pleura or a chronic localization of phlegm and blood in the pleura, both of which could lead on to suppuration, ulceration, and a subsequent full-blown phthisis if they lasted for longer than forty days.

In this case, teasing apart the various lung conditions (including dyspnea or difficulty breathing), and determining how they might mutate, challenged the prognostic skills of the Hippocratic doctors and their successors. Help in this task could be found in *Diseases*, book 2, which delineated the *habitus phthisicus*. That particular people—in this case the tall and thin—tended towards certain diseases—here to phthisis—as a result of their constitution and general physical appearance was part of the holistic conception underpinning humoral medicine. This was a predisposition, not a directly inherited condition, however.

Besides the general body shape, with its long neck, sloping shoulders, and poorly developed chest region, doctors were to look for a reddish hue in the hollows of the eyes, red cheeks, swollen feet, bent finger nails with the pads of flesh lost beneath, emaciation, languor, debility, and hair loss. Listening, they would expect to hear persistent crepitations or crackling during breathing; coughing; and a dull, hoarse voice, perhaps when the patient spoke of pain in the breast and back. When the patient expectorated the sputum was thick, yellow-tinged, and sweet to the taste. This excessively moist, hailstone-like purulent matter gave off a detestable stench when thrown onto the fire. (A useful test: doctors would be throwing sputum onto hot coals for at least the next two thousand years.) Bloody material might also be brought up with the sputum. Concomitantly disturbed bowels and a general swelling below the diaphragm were exceptionally bad signs. Elsewhere reference is made to highly characteristic wing-like shoulder blades; fever with chills; both extreme perspiration and the need to urinate. Much does seem familiar of late-stage pulmonary tuberculosis but it's not an exact fit.

The text *Internal Affections* also listed three kinds of phthisis. The first arose—familiarly now—from an excess of phlegm falling downwards from head to lungs. The second was due to exhaustion and excess: in young males this often referred to venery. The third involved the sufferer initially becoming black and swollen with yellow-tinged skin under the eyes, before a pattern of sputum, cough, fever, and wasting emerged. Patients usually lived for a year with the first form, three years with the second, and as long as nine with the third, when in a wasted state life might yet continue, but the prognosis was very poor. There was therefore much for subsequent medical authorities to work upon. Each tinkered with these composite pictures of phthisics in the light of their own experiences, placing due emphasis on this or that aspect of the consumption and the nature of the original disturbance in the body. Aretaeus of Cappadocia's (*fl.* ?50/100–200 CE) causal triumvirate were abscesses in the lungs, a chronic cough, or haemoptysis. Whatever the details, the causes and course of phthisis were always in the plural.

Galen, the master systematizer of Roman times, ordered, organized, amended, and added to his inheritance of medical knowledge. From a modern vantage point, seeking a continuous trajectory over time, one must look under a multiplicity of Galenic headings—Phthisis, Tabes, Marasmus, Atropy, Phthoe, Phyma, Struma, Haemorrhage, and Hectic Fever—if we want to piece together his understanding of a range of conditions that have been interpreted as tuberculous. For Galen these were separate, if sometimes linked, illnesses. His bequest of the modifier 'hectic' for the fever of phthisis is worth picking out. He described this as a specific disease, which also had the potential to become a phthisis. In contradistinction to other fevers (all of which were diseases, not symptoms of something else, at this time) the heat in a hectic fever was evenly distributed over the body—making it difficult for the patient to detect, the body feeling the same to the touch everywhere—and it did not increase. There was little cough and nothing came up if coughing occurred. Should marasmus (literally withering) occur along with the heat of a hectic fever then phthisis was the likely diagnosis. The seeds of the 'hectic flush' or a 'hectic' beloved by Romantic aesthete male poets and delicate swooning ladies had been sown for the future.

The pathologist Galen commented on the presence of *phûma* or tubercles in phthisics. He was not the first to see these small hard swellings in their lungs and preached the accepted wisdom that these were the result of the bodily disturbances of phthisis, not its cause. In a phthisic's body coction or 'cooking' of the body's juices, such as the excess phlegm in the lungs, was impaired. Tubercles were far from being an exclusive feature of phthisis, however, for this was a general term for hard tumours, which could be abscesses, cancers, water-filled cysts. They occurred in conjunction with a gibbosity or humped spine and its attendant deformities of the associated bones and flesh of the chest. The Greeks knew lung tubercles were found with spinal curvatures, but did not relate the two other than to see their formation as flawed coction in both cases. Bent spines may have been a potent inspiration for the hunchbacked figures in Egyptian and Greek art, but we can be sure of only what was left to posterity not what it represented.

Less dramatic but also easily visible in the living were swellings on the neck: *struma* or strumous disease. Just as 'consumption' was a general term for the wasting of the body and *phûma* for tumour, *struma* implied a tendency to preternaturally hard glands or to a swelling of the glands of the neck and ears. Again there is no neat overlay with the specificity of tubercular lymphatic glands or the more nebulous medieval scrofula. It is reasonable to suppose that among the possible if rare cases of goitre in the Greek world and the chronic inflammations such as mastoiditis, some of these swellings were tuberculous. Rich, inclusive categories of disease functioned in this highly individualized medical cosmology.

What to Do with the Phthisic Patient?

As is so often the case today, Greek texts urged early intervention for the best results. They also cautioned that full-blown cases were likely to end in death. The Hippocratic author of *Internal Affections* knew one way to classify phthisis (in retrospect) was how long his patients survived their symptoms. Nevertheless, doctors did what they could, offering a range of dietary counsel, drugs, lifestyle advice, and surgery. Given the individuality of disease, the more options the better for rebalancing the body. Doctors were required to unite knowledge of therapeutics, past experience of similar afflictions, and their understanding of the patient. Blindly following empirical prescriptions was a greatly inferior medical art.

A change of air or atmosphere could help. This was no two-week pick-me-up in the sun, but the sombre search for a dryer, lighter climate with gentle, favourable winds. Egypt or Libya were popular in the Roman period because they necessitated long journeys from Italy and getting there could in itself be curative. Sea voyages were considered intrinsically healing because of the motion of the boat, including the nausea (purging) and exposure to the sea air, particularly when patients were spitting up blood. If this was beyond the patient's strength (or purse), a sojourn to the nearest coast should be attempted or perhaps a gentle trundle by the sea in a litter could be tried in a severe decline. Should the patient be moribund, the nature of air in the bedroom must be assessed and ventilation keenly attended to.

A change of diet was also recommended. If consumption wasted the body, then according to allopathy, a phthisic's diet called for replenishment. The line between diet and drugs, predominantly herbal at this time, was fluid. Since proper cooking of food in the stomach was an essential component of health, ordinary dietary components—milk, eggs, meat, and wine— took on a more medicinal character under doctor's orders. Milk from various sources—wolves, asses, cows, goats, human breasts—was especially favoured: all to be taken as fresh as possible. Liquid preparations, taken as drinks, might be hyssop and fleawort boiled in sour wine. More solid preparations included combining horehound, pine nuts, parsley, and pepper with honey in a variety of ways. The fumes of ivy could be inhaled. Galen advocated a pound-weight of the mountain squill plant to be steeped for thirty days in strong vinegar, the resulting potion to be taken early each morning when patients had to be brought back from the point of despair. The skill was to know what to give and when.

Bathing was significant—forming in part a useful means of applying external medicines. Myrrh oil infused with a potion of lupines could be applied to the feet, removed, and replaced with butter, the procedure to be repeated three times to draw down the humours. Exercise should be gentle and overexcitement avoided. A successful doctor would also strive for the involvement and commitment of the phthisic to their treatment regime. The patient must remain positive—how else could the doctor be expected to try to combat the inevitable ups and downs during the course of a chronic disease?

Surgical interventions tended to be tried after the diet and drugs had been given a go. If a patient was spitting blood—evidence of excess—venesection, or bleeding, was recommended. Letting blood removed the surplus and cooled the body, helping the impaired lungs do their job. Fasting did the same but while less drastic it was less immediate too, and had to be balanced against the propensity to wasting. Acacia, plantain juice, or other herbal drugs thought to lessen the blood's overabundance might be tried. If the application of glowing hot irons to the chest in order to dry up the superfluous cold and moist humours was too severe, gentler poultices and purges might be tried to the same ends. Modulation of the possible, to meet the needs of the individual, was key.

The diversity and abundance of remedies can be read as evidence for the generalized nature and frequency of consumption. But knowing exactly who and how many suffered from it in antiquity is much harder. One can of course return to the modern analysis of bodily remains using the increasingly sophisticated sampling techniques, but this only answers questions about the epidemiological profile of the much more specific idea of tuberculosis. Qualitative evidence for consumption, while equally bitty, is certainly poignant. The 3rd-century BCE Smyrna funerary stele recounting the long-running misery endured by a 4-year-old child afflicted first in the testicles, then the feet, and finally the intestines—'I, doomed to a sad end…have left the hated consumption as an heritage to those who begat me'—reminds us that not only adults were affected.[12] The Greeks knew that those aged between 18 and 35 were most at risk and included women who were thought to be particularly vulnerable during pregnancy or after amenorrhea—the retention of blood being another potential cause of bodily unbalancing. Such patterns held for centuries—until the 20th century in effect.

There was a firm awareness that consumption could occur in groups of people. What happened apparently was a shared exposure to the correct external conditions of those in a population who had the necessary constitutional predisposition. More directly—but not by way of a living infectious agent— close contact with phthisics could result in a healthy individual developing a phthisis. The risk increased if the victim had stinking breath: an unpleasant and frequent occurrence in those with ulcerated, disintegrating lungs but also other late-stage, chronic, wasting illnesses such as cancers and diabetes. The debate about whether consumption was a contagion, which could be spread in some way from one to another, would swing back and forth across the centuries, a contested matter of opinion. In this, as in many of the other aspects of the identity of consumption, the ideas of the ancient world left a legacy for the tuberculous future.

II

⎯⎯◦≈◦⎯⎯

ALL WITH 'A TOUCH OF CONSUMPTION'?

H istorians do not talk about the Dark Ages any more—
it wasn't so dark after all for the half a millennium or
so that lie between the fall of Rome and the building
of the great Gothic cathedrals. Still, there are some things about
which we still know rather less than we would like to, which
appear to be obscured or opaque. The history of consumption
is one of these. No doubt there is plenty more to be uncovered if
appropriate questions are asked of apposite sources, but much
is annoyingly tentative at the moment. Clear details on who suffered from consumption, how they experienced this suffering,
and exactly how many people it killed are tantalizing but
elusive.

Broadly speaking, second-century Rome was the apogee of
the learned medical knowledge that began with the medics and
natural philosophers of ancient Greece. Thereafter it suffered
along with almost everything else during that broad sweep of
history, the 'decline and fall of the Roman Empire'. The Goths
sacked Rome in 410, and an already fragile administrative structure fragmented, especially in the empire's western half. The
Eastern Empire, run from Constantinople, retained its integrity

for longer, but shrank over time until essentially just the city remained to fall to the Ottomans Turks in 1453, expanding their Islamic empire to the west.

With hindsight, by the mid 5th century the period known as classical antiquity had ended and the Middle Ages begun, lasting for approximately the next thousand years. On the ground, at the time, people adapted as best they could to new levels of uncertainty, including heightened food insecurity and exposure to disease. Under the Romans, daily life, especially for those excluded from urban citizenship, was no picnic, but it was perhaps more ordered than the return to often extreme localism and feudalism which ensued.

Urbanism followed Rome into decay. Not until after the first millennium would towns and cities flourish again as the sophisticated centres they had once been and populations rise to the levels reached before the fall of Rome. Subsistence farming dominated the rural hinterlands. Countryside and metropolis suffered from seriously weakened trade as the market for luxuries, which stimulated commerce, faltered. Interaction with the world beyond the reach of the Roman Empire—modern South Asia and South East Asia—was stymied, especially in the west. Conditions varied across Europe and the Middle East but life was once more 'solitary, poor, nasty, brutish, and short', particularly for the poor and disadvantaged majority both inside and outside the contracted city walls. Circumstances improved in the High Middle Ages (1000–1299), before plague again changed the landscape.

The medieval period is also characterized by the increasing consolidation of the Christian church's power, already under way after Emperor Constantine's conversion in 313, and subsequent legalization of Christianity in the empire. New ideas about the role of health, suffering, illness, and death emerged in an increasingly Christianized Europe. Christianity's attempt at globalization was countermanded by the rise of Islam in the 7th century in the Middle East.

The Roman bureaucratic machine had fostered much, including the Greek-inspired traditions of, and facilities for, learning. In the more unstable times to come luxuries such as expansive scholarship retrenched for practical and ideological reasons. The spirit of questioning, and thereby developing knowledge, was dominated by veneration for existing wisdom, thought by many to be complete. Before the rise of universities as centres of learning in the west in the 11th century, monasteries were the repositories of knowledge. By their laborious copying, monks preserved something of classical learning. Fragile papyri were replaced by more durable parchment, and certain texts translated into Latin.

Further east the Islamic courts offered a different environment for the development of knowledge from the 8th century. Here the classical inheritance was sifted and remixed. For the next 300 years Arabic, Persian, and Syriac translations of Greek medical manuscripts circulated in the Islamic world, as their authors, some Jews and Christians as well as Muslims, tackled the preservation, enhancement, and dissemination of medical knowledge along with the practical realities of treating patients. Their writings formed the basis for another burst of translation, this time into Latin, as part of the expansion of the universities in later medieval and early Renaissance Europe. If books started to replace manuscripts after 1440, when Gutenberg's movable type gradually transformed reading and the dissemination of knowledge in the west (the Chinese had invented movable type several centuries earlier), the contents of medical and scientific texts would also change as the curious looked inside the dead body rather than just inside the covers of a book.

All this means we know much less than we would like to about this period. It would be nice to pinpoint exactly how each of the socio-economic changes—fluxes in living conditions, urbanism, strains imposed by other diseases—affected the incidence and experience of consumption but we cannot: the data are hard to come by for much of this period. Careful sampling of medieval burial grounds looking for bone lesions and latterly aDNA provides some measure of the frequency of the more narrowly defined tuberculosis, but here too absolute values will probably always remain elusive. The tuberculous-disease load in a skeletal sample is only a fraction of the health burden in a population—only 3 to 5 per cent of tuberculosis infections result in bone lesions.[1] Many died of this or something else before such damage occurs, particularly children, whose colossal death rate before the age of 5 brought down life expectancy at birth in the medieval period to below 20 years of age. With the children excluded, the average might go up to the mid-thirties.

Much palaeopathological surveying so far has tended to look for absolute presence, although more recently a population approach has been tried in several locations around the world. In France 2,498 skeletons exhumed from seventeen burial sites of the 4th and 5th centuries, 6th to 8th centuries, and 9th to 11th centuries revealed an inferred rate of infection of 1.2 per cent (29 of 2,498). This figure is thought to be low in comparison with modern rates. Sampling, especially with the relatively small numbers involved here, is inherently vulnerable even with the benefit of appropriate statistical tools. Still, it serves as something of a baseline. Similarly the figures reinforce the expected urban bias, which increases over time. Extrapolating backwards from modern knowledge the increasing population densities, poor housing conditions, a poor diet particularly during the wearisome winter months, and co-infections would all have tended to increase consumption caused by *M. tuberculosis*. As these factors fluctuated throughout the period and across regions, so one would expect to see changes in consumption's epidemiological profile. More people suffering from tuberculosis leads to greater exposure rates and increasing numbers of the sick, but we can only infer—we cannot be sure. It was there when the period began and there when it ended, inexorably rising in demographic significance as the subsequent history testifies.

Reading between the Lines

In the textual history of medicine in the Middle Ages there are a number of places where information on consumptions can be found. A new format—the medical compendium—emerged, varying in length, scope, and anticipated audience. These did not necessarily contain new material but presented what was already known in a neat encyclopedic mode. Brevity was useful for those wishing to memorize the contents and some came to be written and illustrated in a deliberately mnemonic style. Where facilities for medical learning faltered most severely, the newer texts emphasized treatment as part of a do-it-yourself domestic medicine. Later on women's recipe books, digests of the domestic economy, often contained prescriptions for home use.

Texts aimed at practitioners rather than theoreticians removed some of the intriguing uncertainties and ambiguities of the originals. At the elite end Caelius Aurelianus (*fl.* late 4th or early 5th century) Latinized and perhaps emended the earlier

work of the Greek Methodist Soranus (*fl.* 100). Soranus' sect
largely eschewed theory and sought to treat what was observable. He had divided diseases into acute and chronic categories.
The latter included the long-drawn-out consumptions, befitting
their gradual wasting qualities, but acute episodes of bleeding
from the lungs for instance, seen as separate afflictions, were
among the acute conditions. Aurelianus' extremely useful
rendition of *Acute and Chronic Diseases* was used throughout the
medieval period.

Isaac Judaeus (*c.*840–932), a court physician who worked in
Cairo and Tunisia, codified his understanding of consumption
differently, devoting part three of his five-part *Book on Fevers* to
'hectic fever or consumption'. Part one discussed the general
nature of fever—an unnatural heat—as opposed to the natural
or innate heat characteristic of, and necessary for, living bodies.
Part two concentrated on 'one day fever', part four on acute
fevers and part five on purulent or putrid fevers. In comparison
with the Galenic tradition and Avicenna (980–1037), the most
celebrated exponent of Islamic medicine, Isaac's conception of
consumption was more unified. He may have made less of ulceration in the lungs (important to the classical authors) and the
drenching night-sweats (a key descriptor in the modern tubercular lexicon) but his text served as a 'clinical companion to its
subject'.[2] It was well received among his Arabic colleagues.

Isaac wrote with his elite patients of northern Africa in mind.
Some of his dietary recommendations—pomegranate juice, an
astringent to help the diarrhoea—would have been impossible
to fulfil in 9th-century northern Europe. Likewise advice on
which part of the house a patient should spend the day in and
where to sleep at night also reflected the warm, dry, sunny
climate in which he and his patients lived. The surrounding air

was particularly important because this was what the patient had most contact with. He specified the necessity for the right type of cooling breeze, a northern exposure, sheltered from the heat and hot winds. Clothes by their 'very nature' were to be 'cool, fresh, soft and pleasant to the touch…washed and scented'. 'Spray the face liberally with rose-water and then fan the patient', he intoned, for the doctor must leave 'no stone unturned in trying to prevent any dissolution occurring in the body'.[3] It sounds heavenly if one were not suffering from consumption. Isaac's recommendations would have made sensible reading some nine or ten centuries later when doctors sent their consumptive patients south for the climate.

He opened by focusing on the differential diagnosis of a patient's decline, sorting out the natural (old age) from the sickly and then delineating the kinds associated with illness. As we would expect from an author basing himself on classical texts, there was not one but three kinds of hectic fever which increased in severity—measured by the degree of heat, its duration, and the physicians' ability to offer effective treatment. Intense, protracted heat destroyed not just the new moisture, which the body created to build itself but the 'essential moisture', which in humoral physiology held together the body and protected its organs. By this stage no treatment would work. He compared the effects of this fever to that of sun on wood or stone: long exposed to the harsh rays, it is reduced to an ash-like state, a graphic description of the extreme emaciation of end-stage tuberculosis.

He discussed the relationship of hectic fevers with other illness, which might precede or succeed them. We might see these as stages along the path of tuberculosis or they could be unrelated symptoms; at this distance one cannot be sure. A hectic combined with a putrid fever was a serious threat and hard to manage; it can perhaps be equated with our understanding of advanced tuberculosis of the lungs, where there is extensive open tissue damage. The two kinds of fever required incompatible treatments. Isaac relied upon his own skills to find a combination that would cool, moisten, and soothe simultaneously. He claimed he could find no precedent in the accounts available to him. The extensive list of prescriptions closing *On Consumption*—several of his own devising—tell how Isaac would treat the various forms of tussis (cough) and diarrhoea a patient might present. For a haemoptysis—occurring when the secretions of the chest were sufficiently pungent to burn through the veins in the chest and cause them to burst—he listed syrups and plasters. He noted that these were also useful in non-consumptives who were spitting blood—a reminder that symptomatology was essentially all. He didn't follow Galen's advice to prescribe venesection.

Isaac was silent on the infectiousness of consumption, although from the 9th century onwards, other Arabic writers began to discuss the concept of *i'dā* or transmissibility. This broad concept could mean infection, contagion, and hereditability. By the 10th century Al-Majūsī (d. *c*.994), who shared Isaac's interest in fevers, classified consumption, or *sill*, as a transmissible disease in his comprehensive medical compendium. Here he discussed the risks of keeping company and chatting with a consumptive, specifically inhaling the 'evil vapour' arising from their body, reinforcing the views of various of the classical authors who also warned against such contact. The merits of infection and/or contagion and/or heredity would continue to ebb and flow.

Other sources included texts that followed the popular head-to-toe format, describing illnesses (cause, diagnosis, prognosis, and treatment) by body region. Sections on the chest area—housing the potentially ulcerating, consumptive lungs—were often the shortest.[4] Knowledge of the mechanisms of breathing and lung anatomy was relatively limited. At this time (indeed until the 17th century) while known to be functionally different, the lungs were believed to be structurally similar to the liver, spleen, and pancreas. Galen's physiology of the three pneumata or spirits—natural (associated with the liver), vital (associated with the heart), and animal (associated with the brain)—had raised the question of whether inhaled air was more than a mere cooling agent. Did it act as a kind of food for the organs, something tangible brought into the body by the lungs, and what implications did this have for explaining lung function? The established cooling function tended to dominate and anyway this was the sort of refinement that the more basic compendia omitted.

Phthisis nestled among an apparently eclectic range of other conditions afflicting the chest area—eclectic because we now tend to group by cause, rather than by location, regardless of cause. However, several of these illnesses did involve the excess of phlegm implicated in phthisis: a commonality to be teased apart by the doctor when attending his patient at the bedside. The modern tuberculosis-spotter would rightly suggest some of these could have had a tubercular element or been symptoms of this disease, but as in the classical period, they remained distinct entities. William of Brescia (1250–1326) included chapters on cough, phthisis, pneumonia, spitting of blood, and asthma in his *Manual of Practice for Every Disease from Head to Foot*. Bernard of Gordon's *Lily of Medicine* (written 1303–5) had a few more: quinsy (sore throat), problems with the uvula (flap of skin in the throat), hoarseness, cough, phthisis ('ulcer of the lung with consumption of the whole body'), splitting blood, empyema, asthma, pleurisy, pneumonia, heart tremor, syncope (fainting), diseases of the breasts. As in the classical period, we infer the ubiquity of consumptions from their inclusion in a wide range of medical texts. Though in the encyclopedic era, with its arranging and rearranging, what started out in the medical literature mostly remained there.

Beyond Europe Chinese medical texts from the Sui and Tang dynasties (6th to 10th centuries) included detailed information on the treatment of phthisis indicating familiarity with the disease. By the 12th century in an aptly titled text—'The Disease which Changes a Living Being into a Corpse'—Daoist priests described the influence of deviant airs (*qi*), and infectious agents—animalculae—to which a weakened or exhausted person was particularly vulnerable. A body full of vitality had no space within it for disease-inducing winds to enter. In a weakened one, the contagious elements evolved in the patient's body during the course of the disease and at the end of their sixth stage became especially infectious. Sometimes read as a pre-germ theory 'germ theory', the Chinese ideas of infectiousness were rooted in a very different conception of the body and its relationship to the wider world.

Just as Greek and Islamic medical texts moved around the world following the ebb and flow of the political world, so too did Chinese medical knowledge. Medieval Japanese rulers imported elite medical knowledge and doctors from China and Korea as part of a deliberate transfer of technology to bolster their power and reputation. Japanese doctors of this period thus looked for, and found, cases of consumption according to their own rules.

Despite its persistent presence consumption apparently didn't press for attention. There was some serious competition.

The drama and intensity of the acute infectious diseases (as we would think of them) often swamped such chronic conditions. Rhazes (c.865–925/932), one of the great Islamic authors, thought it important to elucidate the difference between chickenpox and smallpox. Smallpox was of course a major cause of death while those lucky enough to survive were immune, safe from further attacks if scarred. St Anthony's fire (chronic gangrenous ergot poisoning from contaminated rye) swept across Europe. When there wasn't enough to eat, typhus—the famine disease par excellence—carried off large numbers. And everyone knows that the Middle Ages were also the years of the great plague epidemics, most famously the Black Death peaking in Europe between 1347 and 1351. Among the chronic diseases, leprosy repelled. Ancient and medieval leprosy was a more inclusive diagnosis than modern ideas of the spectrum caused by *M. leprae* (also known today as Hansen's disease) but it included these conditions. The highly visible disfigurements and disablements of leprosy caught the eye and imagination, especially the Christian imagination. What then of consumption?

Getting It in the Neck:
The Special Case of Scrofula

A special visibility was afforded to its glandular form—characterized by swollen or diseased neck glands. Scrofulas, according to the 5th-century author and translator Cassius Felix, could be 'hard round bodies implanted in sinews, arteries, veins and muscular membranes', which 'when they develop in the glandular areas on both sides of the throat … show up painfully just like the swollen neck of a sow'. These were difficult to cure. The swellings could also be free-floating, under the skin rather than adhered; found in the 'glandular regions, like the neck, armpit, and groin'; tending to multiply 'like swine' and amenable to treatment by medicine or surgery.[5] Scrofula came to have other names and meanings—the royal disease, the King's Evil—and a specialized cure—the 'royal touch' or simply 'touching' or 'stroking'. Scrofula and scrofulous consumption, when wasting accompanied the swellings, thus became a distinctively visible form of our disease in this period. By the early modern period scrofula was sufficiently perceptible and repellent for 'scrofulous' to become a term of abuse, characteristic of the lowest, smelliest echelons of the despised urban poor.

For the Roman medical writers the 'royal sickness' had meant a jaundice-like condition caused by an excess of yellow bile, but unrelated to swollen neck glands. By the 4th century an alternative meaning—derived via the Christian church fathers—referred to wasting diseases, consuming the body in an offensive manner, sometimes involving worms, and including the broadly defined leprosy. These two non-scrofulous definitions of the royal sickness ran side by side. At some point in the 11th and 12th centuries in Anglo-Saxon England the second wasting/scabrous definition was applied also to swellings, eruptions, and carbuncles which could appear anywhere on the face and body.

William of Malmesbury was able to write in the 12th century of isolated reports of miraculous cures following attendance at royal tombs and the touch of Edward the Confessor (c.1033–1066). In France sufferers from scrofula, struma, and other skin diseases had a patron saint, Marculf or Marcoul at Corbigny. By the 13th century, scrofulas were definitely part of the royal sickness and the populations of England and France were invited to come for the royal cure in the same way they attended religious sites and tombs for holy blessing. In his *Compendium medicinae* (*c.*1250) Gilbert the Englishman linked the 'royal disease' with scrofulas and glands, commenting seemingly without guile that it was named the 'king's disease', because 'kings cure this disease'.

Having uncertainly become part of the royal disease, it is not absolutely clear why scrofula (or *écrouelles* for the French) eventually came to dominate the illnesses treated by the interrelated royal families of England and France from the 13th century to the reign of Britain's Queen Anne (r. 1702–14) and the French Revolution (1789). The ascendancy may be partly by default. For some learned medics, including Gilbert, the association of the original Roman meaning of excess yellow bile faded away. So too did the presence of the leprous as they were hived off into lazarettos, befitting the moral corruption apparent in their displeasing appearance.

But why would the monarch be interested in touching, however briefly, their rather disgustingly diseased subjects? The answer lies partly in the claims of a divine entitlement to rule. Newly resurgent kings sought to bolster power among rivals for the crown (Edward IV and Richard III's antagonists claimed neither could cure and hence were illegitimate squatters). In France they also wished to manoeuvre into a position of dominance over the church. If kingship was a divine office following the anointment with holy oil at the coronation, kings could heal and such a demonstration of healing ensured the incumbent's credentials. The church countered by claiming only properly holy monarchs could heal and suggested that those who had lapsed morally lost their thaumaturgical powers. Touching also proved to be a useful device for giving a semblance of accessibility to the wider population. Better for the king to get on with it then.

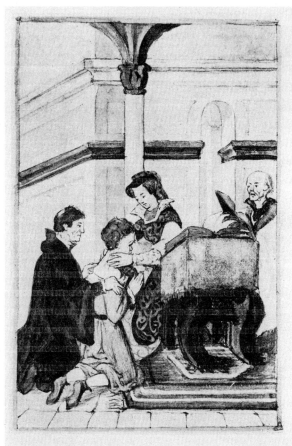

QUEEN MARY TOUCHES A SCROFULOUS BOY
From *Queen Mary's Manual.* (Library of the Roman Catholic
Cathedral, Westminster.)

2. England's Queen Mary (r. 1553–8) was keen to practise the Royal Touch
against scrofula to prove her right to the throne. She urged those she touched
never to be parted from the gold coin or 'touch piece' she gave them at the ceremony. (*Wellcome Library, London*)

What of the patients? What could they expect from their innate belief in royalty's supernatural powers? During Edward the Confessor's inaugural 'touching' he had anointed the face of his young female patient with water. She was 'suffering from an infection of the throat and of those parts under the jaw ... which had so disfigured her face with an evil smelling disease that she could hardly speak to anyone without great embarrassment', but had dreamed that Edward could cure her. He made the sign of the cross, and proceeded to knead the diseased areas of her face and neck 'with his holy hand and drew out the pus' plus worms and blood until 'with his healing hand he had brought out all that noxious disease. Then he ordered her to be fed daily at the royal expense until she should be fully restored to health.'[6] Such careful, ad hoc care as Edward reputedly offered was replaced by a rather more streamlined version as touching became the increasingly institutionalized cure for a newly reformulated royal disease.

The records of the gifts of alms provide useful numerical details of those seeking relief. These records refer to those who successfully made the cut from the still larger crowds who gathered outside the court at the appointed time, usually in association with the major festivals of the church. All of which in reality can be but a tiny fraction of those who needed the cure. Officers of the court (later including the king's physicians) selected those they felt would most likely benefit. Edward I touched 627 people in 1277, 197 in 1284, 1,736 in 1290 (the highest figure from the royal accounts), and 983 in 1300; Edward II touched 214 in 1316, and Edward III ranged from 10 in 1336/7 to 885 in 1338/40. The monarchs touched when they could, when the court was temporarily settled. In between, there was travel, warfare, and other duties to fit in so variations in the numbers need to be read with this in mind.[7] Monarchs touched the face of those who knelt before them and 'signed'—made the sign of the cross—over them. The English tended to be more liturgical than the French, although in 1314, on his deathbed Philip IV recited the secret formula to his son and successor Louis X.

The traditional gift of alms was also significant. Such charity was initially intended to help defray travel expenses. Touchingly, parishes would raise money to send patients on their way (attendees would be fed and temporarily housed at the expense of the monarch). Edward III upgraded the original penny to a new coin—the Angel—worth 6 shillings. These 'touch pieces' become talismanic. Royal, supernatural relics that fetched a reasonable second-hand value, they also reminded of the cure's time-frame. Immediate, miraculous relief from suffering would have been nice, but the scrofulous understood that their cure may well occur at some point in the future. For those who did indeed have tubercular adenitis such a delayed response could be part of its natural history of waxing and waning. Or perhaps the later fate of 'the scholastic Michel Martin' (d. 1657) awaited many: 'He had been sent to France for the healing of his scrofula by laying on of hands from the most Christian King, and come back cured to Portugal; but he then succumbed to another disease and fell victim to a slow consumption': a scrofula portending to an ultimately more widespread tuberculosis infection?[8]

Famous as the cure became, eventually finding its way from French and English authors into the international medical literature of the 16th century, touching was not the only remedy. There was the usual hierarchy of procedures. Bernard of Gordon suggested: 'As a last resort recourse must be had to the surgeon, or if not we must approach the king.' Similarly John of Gaddesden (c.1280–1349): 'If all remedies prove ineffective, let the patient go to the King and be touched and blessed by him, in the very last resort, if everything else has proved ineffective let him hand himself over to the surgeon.'[9]

Obviously the healing cult associated with Christian monarchs had no place in Islamic lands. Here, as well as the traditional remedies of antiquity, surgery was pursued. Indeed advancements subsequently found their way back to the Latin west. Surgeons were aware of the potentially disfiguring effects of cutting out the swellings, and authors of surgical texts bore this in mind when providing instructions. Popular advice books also contained helpful remedies. Since most treatments for scrofula, indeed for all consumptions, would have taken place within the family or community the ready availability of ingredients was important. Common snails, specifically white- or grey-shelled ones, were to be beaten to a paste in a mortar and the plaster-like residue applied to the sores, once a day: what better use for this otherwise molluscan bane of the gardener?

Bubbling Under, about to Burst Forth: Consumption in the Age of Leprosy, Plague, and Beyond

The scrofulous began their queue for the touch in a period when urban populations, movement, and trade began to expand again. Greater numbers and movement brought new controls by the church and local burgesses. Long a source of stigma, the Third Lateran Council of 1179 established formal requirements for the housing, church attendance, and burial of lepers, differentiated gradually from the merely scrofulous. This resulted in their formal segregation outside the city walls after a funeral mass and symbolic burial. Those not incarcerated in asylums or lazarettos were required to wear identifying clothing and carry a wooden clapper to warn of their approach. Such regulations persisted through the peak of the European leprosy epidemic of the 12th and 13th centuries. Cases were still reported in England and Scotland during the next two centuries, but by the 16th century leprosy had virtually disappeared in Europe except for the northern regions of Scandinavia.

Historical epidemiologists interested in the changing disease profile of later medieval and early modern Europe found that the declining cases of leprosy were subsequently followed by a rise in the incidence of pulmonary tuberculosis. By the time London's bills of mortality were being published in the 17th century, consumption (outside the plague years) accounted for some 20 per cent of deaths. As we know, consumption did not equate exactly with tuberculosis but it remained essentially the same recognizable entity throughout this period. Was there a causal connection then, over a longish period? Did the church's strengthening power to control the lives of the leprous enhance the spread of tuberculosis among their number through confinement and the other forms of social marginalization? Did tuberculosis come to the fore after the epidemics of plague in the 14th century had emptied out the lazarettos?

Reports from late 19th- and 20th-century leprosaria have provided some general information, which allows for possible historical analogies. In many of these institutions, tuberculosis was the most significant complication and it was associated with the attendant overcrowding and poor hygiene. Perhaps something more specific was happening too? Given the interrelatedness of the causal bacteria of leprosy and bacteria what about an immunological overlap between the two conditions? Did exposure to M. tuberculosis, which resulted in a latent infection, protect individuals from contracting leprosy? Or were the leprous in fact more susceptible to the effects of latent tuberculosis because their compromised immune systems left them particularly open to the development of the full-blown disease at a more rapid rate? Both immunological scenarios could result in fewer cases of leprosy but at the price of an increasing presence of tuberculosis over a period of several centuries.

Comparative palaeopathology and aDNA analysis have been used to provide some suggestive answers. Recently samples of bone from sites in Israel (1st century), Egypt (4th century), Sweden (10th–13th centuries) and Hungary (10th–11th/14th–16th centuries) were tested for M. tuberculosis and M. leprae DNA and some 40 per cent of the sample showed the presence of both.[10] The ability to recover aDNA from the bones is interpreted as evidence of a disseminated and active infection rather than a latent, quiescent, and potentially protective one. Investigating the immunological effects of leprosy (particularly the rapidly advancing form) indicates that the body is rendered more vulnerable to attack by tuberculosis bacteria. Such impairment is exceptionally acute in the 22 per cent of the population who share a certain genetic defect, which makes them less able to cope with the predations of these microbes. In this scenario, tuberculosis was not protecting against leprosy but accelerating the deaths of those with both diseases. Over a couple of hundred years then, this may indeed have helped empty out the leprosaria. Moreover, the level of exposure to M. tuberculosis revealed by such studies, if extrapolated to the wider population, could be indicative of a considerable underlying rate of tuberculosis.

Studies of the burden of chronic disease afflicting the northern Italian cities, the places that led medieval Europe into the

Renaissance, provides further evidence for such an emerging disease profile. Scrutiny of the Medici family's medical histories from 15th-century Florence reveals several cases of underlying tubercular infections, in addition to those who were explicitly consumptive. More systematically, the death registers maintained to warn of an impending epidemic of plague (epidemic diseases, especially plague, struck on average three times in twenty years) inform about occurrence of chronic diseases during life. The *Necrologi* of 15th-century Milan are particularly good. In many cases cause of death data are supplemented by details of the symptoms leading up to death and age at death. The records of predecease symptoms help us decide how much of the broader diagnostic category of consumption we might tentatively ascribe to pulmonary tuberculosis. Age at death reveals a peak of phthisis deaths occurring in early adulthood and is consistent with lingering childhood exposures or reactivations of latent infections. A similar reactivation process was also at work for the large numbers of the over-sixties swept away by 'catarrh'. In the northwest of France at Plougonver in Brittany, good mid-17th-century records list respiratory illness as the leading cause of death. While due credit must be given to the deadliness of pneumonias and influenza among the acute respiratory diseases, tuberculosis would have added to this burden and accounted for a large number by itself.

Outside of the flashpoints of acute epidemic diseases, consumption was quietly and inexorably becoming the most significant cause of adult mortality in the 17th century. It was increasingly recognized that unlike the sudden acute illness and death it at least allowed its sufferers the time to prepare for death materially and spiritually. As such it edged towards what church and patient both might like to think of as a good death, physical suffering aside. What then did the doctors make of it, besides counting the dead?

Tubercles to the Fore?

Beginning in the Renaissance and gathering pace in the early modern period, there was a new quest to understand the natural world, including the human body. There was a new interest in form—in the normal and then pathological anatomy. Similarly for function, experiment joined with new ways of thinking about how the body operated in health and disease. There were calls to revise clinical practice by returning to the bedside to gather information as the Hippocratics had done. Opportunities grew to exploit the newer chemical remedies or the new plant materials that arrived at home, products of exploration and increasingly globalized sea trading.

There was no immediate abandonment of existing clinical medicine, but a relatively static humoral pathology would be progressively challenged by new ideas derived from chemistry and physics. Bodies were opened more frequently and, by some, more systematically. In the lungs of consumptives there was much to be seen (and smelt) including pus, larger regions of destroyed tissue forming cavities, and smaller swellings or tubercles. There was nothing new in merely observing the presence of tubercles: the ancients had seen them, Galen referred to them, and anyone who had copied or encyclopedized in the succeeding centuries would have repeated it, even if they hadn't seen it for themselves.

Tubercles featured in the necropsies of one of the progressive leaders of Netherlands medicine, the anatomist, chemist, and clinician Franciscus Sylvius (1614–72). Sylvius was one of the new iatrochemists who conceived of all the processes in the living body such as digestion and emotion, as a perpetual series of balanced chemical reactions, principally the interactions of acids and alkalis with their ensuing effervescence and fermentation. The liquids (humours) were still pre-eminent for Sylvius, with blood as the most important. Disease in this Sylvian model resulted from imbalanced, acrimonious reactions with either too much acid or too much alkali and it was within this framework that he explained abnormal fluids and morbid appearances in the solid parts of the body. He used the same rationale of rebalancing the acids and alkalis as the basis for his treatments. He was able to test some of his ideas in his laboratory, but also relied upon theoretical speculation.

Sylvius came to various conclusions about tubercles and consumption. He is often lauded for his modernism, in calling for a greater specificity in diagnosis. He recommended that phthisis be used only to describe those whose wasting was subsequently shown to involve tubercles in the lung (although we must remember that tubercle was a general term for swellings of various kinds, not the specific lesion it would become). He considered the tubercles to be ulcers, bound by a thin membrane, because when cut in section they contained pussy material. Aware that they came in various sizes, he did not distinguish between smaller tubercles and larger purulent cavities; they were both to be found in the same disease of phthisis.

Sylvius thought the tubercles might begin as abnormally developed glands in the tissues of the lungs; in health these glands were present but too small to be seen. Sylvius endorsed the two recently discovered body systems: William Harvey's circulation of the blood and Thomas Bartholin's circulation of lymph. His interest in the lymphatic system may have directed his attention to the swellings he found in various lymph glands and ducts in the neck, thorax, and abdomen but he did not relate these extrapulmonary tubercles to phthisis.

Richard Morton (1637–98) believed consumption sufficiently common among his patients in the city of London to write an all-encompassing text on this disease at its most expansive. Highly regarded on its publication in Latin (1689) and then in English translation (1694), *Phthisiologia* found a ready readership among clinicians and the research-minded in the years to come. Exhaustively piecing together the stories of his consumptive patients during his years in practice in the city of London, he confided grimly, 'I cannot sufficiently admire that anyone, at least after he comes to the flower of youth, can die without a touch of consumption.'[11] He abhorred the unhealthy state of London's smoky air, like the diarist John Evelyn who wrote:

> And what is all this, but that Hellish and dismall Cloud of SEACOALE?…so universally mixed with the otherwise wholesome and excellent Aer, that her Inhabitants breathe nothing but an impure and thick Mist accompanied with a fuliginous and filthy vapour which renders them obnoxious to a thousand inconveniences corrupting the Lungs, and disordering the entire habits of their Bodies; so that Cattharrs, Phthisicks; Coughs and Consumptions rage.[12]

Morton echoed earlier comments saying he could have done more for his patients had they come to him sooner. Too many, he lamented, either ignored their coughs and fevers or worse still wasted money and time in the hands of a quack, old woman, or mere apothecary until a minister for the 'future Salvation of their Souls, and the Advice of a Lawyer about making their Last Will' would prove more efficacious.[13]

Morton divided his consumptions into three main types. The first were general consumptions, or atrophies, and included nervous, diabetic, dropsical affections and those afflicting nursing women who had overexpended their energy producing milk, particularly when their own appetite was poor. 'Milk is nothing but the Nutritious Juice continually separated from the Mass of Blood by the Glandules of the Breasts', so if this extraction of the juice went on too long, the blood would become impoverished.[14] Impoverished blood would lead to a hectical heat in the blood, spirits, and frame of the body and atrophy would ensue. Paradoxically he reported that in women of a consumptive disposition breast-feeding could act as a cure, citing among his examples his 'most dear wife'. His reasoning became clear, however: in these predisposed cases a nursing woman's appetite was stimulated by the continual separation of the nutritious juice. If she ate enough while she gave suck, the increased flow of nutritious juices to the milk would allow room in her body for a greater quantity of new rich chyle (produced after the digestion of food) to be absorbed. Such augmented blood 'does conduce more to the Cure of the Consumptive Disposition, than all the Medicines in the World', he claimed.[15]

Morton's second and third types of consumption were both an 'original Consumption of the lungs', either a 'consumption of the lungs' which was 'a Consumption of the whole Body with a Fever, proceeding first from an ill Affection, and at length an Exulceration of the Lungs' or a 'Secondary, and Symptomatical, whenever the Lungs receive any great Injury from preceding Distempers'.[16] Taking the last first, these 'distempers' could be a predisposing disease in the lungs or elsewhere so there could be a scrofulous, scorbutical, asthmatical, hysterical, or hypochondriacal consumption. Melancholy might precede consumption, as could spitting of blood; suppression of the menses; the French pox; gout; fevers such as scarlet fever, small-pox, and measles; 'pleurisie' (pleurisy), or 'peripneumony' (pneumonia). Even the unintentional swallowing of foreign materials—'Nails, pins and other things, that flip down into the Lungs as People laugh…unless they are quickly cough'd up again, they prick the Lungs, and cause a lanciating [piercing or pricking] Pain, from whence a spitting of Blood, Ulcers, and a Consumption are wont to proceed.'[17]

Morton gave a detailed account of just such a case history. A young man working at his trade of whiting (plastering) acci-dentally let three nails into his lungs. He immediately suffered a spell of harsh coughing and spitting blood, but the nails remained lodged. After several months of relatively good health broken only by a dry cough he decided to marry. On his wed-ding night he was struck with great pain, spasms, coughing, and fever. Morton prescribed bleeding and external and internal treatments to soothe the cough, promote expectoration of phlegm, and control the fever. But although the patient's symp-toms eased, it was but a temporary respite: 'he grew every Day weaker, and at length from a Universal Colliquation, he dyed plainly of a Consumption within the space of a Month or five Weeks.'[18]

Morton described an 'original' consumption of the lungs as 'the most famous Consumption, and that which is called so by Way of Eminence'.[19] It was in this kind of consumption that Syl-vius' tubercles featured and Morton described its progress through three stages or degrees, each more severe for the patient and more difficult for the physician to treat. He had an extensive list of predisposing causes ranging from blocked evacuations of any kind, morbid emotions, too many late nights, and too much studying, overindulgence in meats and liquors, a hereditary disposition, an infection: 'For this Distemper, like a contagious Fever, does infect those that lie with the sick Person with a certain Taint.'[20]

What tied all these disparate forms together was that the body's imbalanced juices in some way caused them, just as they featured in the breast-feeding consumptive mother and as a consequence of the inhalation of nails. In the original consumption the injury was immediately to the lungs where the 'sharp or malignant *Serum* or Water of the Blood being separated by the soft and glandulous Substance of the Lungs, does stuff, inflame, and at length also exulcerate the Lungs themselves, which is the immediate Cause of this Distemper'.[21] It was this same process which led to the formation of the tubercles.

Such swellings could appear everywhere in the body, but they were particularly common in the lungs, he said, because of the structural propensity of the lungs to 'suck in and retain the humours' in its 'small Bladders and Vessels' and their constant movement during respiration.[22] Indeed they were so common he thought that if it were not for their natural tendency to go as quickly as they came (or be helped by the doctor's art) 'a Consumption of the Lungs would necessarily be the common Plague of Mankind'.[23] Benign tubercles faded without causing disease; malignant tubercles ripened, hardened, and destroyed the natural tone of the tissue; became inflamed and ulcerated; and served as the immediate cause of a consumption of the lungs.

Morton advised a range of symptomatic treatments, including the new Peruvian Bark (the source of quinine) for the attendant fever. He favoured letting blood and the use of long-established soothing pectorals (drugs for the chest), linctuses, and lozenges for the cough. Opiates had an important role, as did soothing balsamic medicines.

Exhaustive though Morton's prescriptions were, the final word in consumptive cure in the 17th century must go to the 'English Hippocrates', Thomas Sydenham (1624–89). He also employed bleeding, purging, and balsamics:

> But of all the remedies for phthisis, long and continued journeys on horseback bear the bell; in respect to which it must be noted, that if the patient be past the prime of life, more exercise of the sort in question must be taken than if he were a youth or boy. Bark is no surer a cure for ague, than riding for phthisis.[24]

Sydenham's words were sharp and to the point. He was one of the first to recognize that despite the individuality of humoral medicine even in its new chemical and mechanical guises, there were specific diseases. His confidence stemmed from his experience with the bark and ague. Regardless of their disposition, anyone who suffered from ague or malaria (and many did in 17th-century southern Britain) benefited from a dose of the bark, their cure resulting from the quinine it contained. He was making a similar argument for the specificity of phthisis.

Sydenham, though, was just one voice among many. There was less of a consensus, more a rich maelstrom of ideas and certainly a lot of coughing, spitting, flushing, fever, and death. Specificity had more of a chance with the revised notion of the tubercle in consumption's long 18th century.

III

ᕙᕗ

TUBERCLES, AIRS, WATERS,
AND PLACES

ven in cold weather with a relatively fresh corpse, opening the bodies of those who had died of a consumption
would have been unpleasant. An already wasted frame
was rendered skeletal by the disease's final depredations. If the
chest were cut into, the lungs were often found adhered to the
surrounding tissues, and could not be separated without considerable force. The cavity in which they sat might contain various liquids: an 'aqueous humour', some 'sanious fluid'—a thin
fetid pus tinged with blood, or the full-blown residues of suppuration in which bits of tissue floated. The lobes of the lungs
frequently appeared shrunken, contracted, and hardened. The
first incision could release a waft of foul air and reveal a disgust-
ing mass of necrosing tissue: there would be little left to see. It
would be as if 'the lungs themselves are melted down by suppuration, and pour'd out into the thorax'.[1] The stench alone pre-
cluded going further. It wasn't easy to know what had occurred
before and what after death.

Despite its disagreeableness, those driven to understand the
effects of disease upon the body pursued this course. Among
the abscesses, empyema, livid pleura, and destroyed lung tissue,

anatomists consistently reported the presence of swellings or tubercles in some consumptives. In consumption's long 18th century, ending with René Laennec's work published in 1819, the tubercles came of age. They were transformed from a common post-mortem finding in consumptives to a specific, pathognomonic sign, detectable in the body during life, using the stethoscope. While anatomists braved the interior of the body, doctors continued to diagnose and prescribe, and patients to endure the 'longest and most dangerous of all chronic diseases'.[2]

'Fill'd with Many Tubercles'

One of the 18th century's leading anatomists, the Italian Giovanni Battista Morgagni (1682–1771) spent much of his long career at the University of Padua, where he taught, practised medicine, and above all dissected. Morgagni's life's work was to describe the symptoms observed during life and the post-mortem findings after death. This encompassed his own patients, those of his contemporaries with whom he corresponded, and the long dead, who featured in past works he read and mulled over. All were reviewed and integrated into his landmark text *On the Seats and Causes of Diseases Investigated by Anatomy* (1761). It was a vast project drawing on the continuity of medical knowledge up to the mid 18th century. Yet Morgagni only once reported personally opening a consumptive body; as a young man, he feared the possible threat to his health, and when old he feared for that of his students. His contribution should not be judged by this statistic. He was well aware of the epidemiological significance of consumption and pondered the role of the tubercle.

Morgagni worked through the body from head to foot, describing the diseases affecting each region. Arriving at the thorax, he reported on the location and condition of tubercles in diseased lungs. Some had claimed that tubercles predominated in the upper part of the lung, but Morgagni tended towards the view that these swellings were just as likely to be found 'promiscuously' throughout the lungs—sometimes they were literally 'fill'd with many tubercles'.[3] So, position was not suggestive. He outlined their structure. Tubercles (as observed with the naked eye) seemed to begin as insensate solids, resembling the normal appearance of 'conglobate' or ball-like glands. Subsequently various kinds of matter were found within the tubercle's coat: pus; a honey-like substance; 'steatomatous' (fatty or suet-like) material; and a soft, pasty, or poultice-like stuff. He explained this range of fillings by reference to the variability of the disease in individual patients. Each had its own cause—similar to Morton's long list of secondary, 'symptomatical' consumptions—and each acted on a patient's personal constitution. His aim was to provide a comprehensive picture of what might be seen, case history by case history.

When it came to assessing the tubercle's role in originating consumptions, Morgagni moved beyond mere observation and invoked the time-honoured if updated humoral theory of the 18th century. He explained how the acrid humour, thrown off by the tubercle, stagnated and then eroded the substance of the lungs. Once this began, the erosion spread and larger cavities appeared as Sylvius had already indicated. There was a recognizable process, but not an exclusive relationship between tubercles, cavitations, and consumptions. Morgagni gave two reasons why. First, following tradition everyone knew that 'pulmonary consumption may be brought on from other causes besides suppurated tubercles'.[4] Secondly, the morbid appearances of pus and ulcers, bound in some kind of a coat, were not necessarily the remains of tubercles.

Morgagni wondered about the similarity between tubercles and glands: were the pathological swellings in the lungs the same as the glands he saw surrounding the windpipe (trachea) and its branches (bronchia) within the lungs? Naturally small in health, these glands could increase in size too, but was this necessarily pathological? Here he was bound to admit that he simply had not performed enough comparative dissections between the sick and the healthy to be very confident. He was more certain about Morton's assertions on the relationship between glands, tubercles, and consumption of the lungs. He quoted with approval Morton's observation that the scrofulous 'who are frequently subject to glandular tumours in other parts of the body, are frequently affected with tubercles of the same kind, in the lungs'. Morton also advised that the most telling sign of a scrofulous consumption was the presence of 'glandulous tumours...on the external surface of the body'.[5] Such a linkage based on specific morbid appearances was pregnant for future consideration.

'No Morbid Appearance So Common'

An erudite meta-analysis of pathological anatomy past and present, Morgagni's was a magisterial book, but one of his sharpest disciples, Matthew Baillie (1761–1823) wanted more on the morbid appearances and less of the chat surrounding each case history. Much of this was unspecific and tended towards irrelevancy, he thought. Baillie was part of a distinguished medical family, a nephew of the brothers William and John Hunter.

The Hunters were movers and shakers in surgery, medicine, midwifery, and comparative and pathological anatomy in the second half of the 18th century. All three moved south from their native Scotland, Baillie joining his uncles in London in 1780. Here he walked the wards of St George's Hospital and attended William's Great Windmill Street anatomy school, which he ran after Hunter's death in 1783.

Like Morgagni, Baillie produced a comprehensive text on pathological anatomy, *The Morbid Anatomy of Some of the Most Important Parts of the Human Body* (1793). Where Morgagni was prolix, Baillie was concise. Clinically astute through his practice and hospital teaching, he concentrated on presenting a résumé of diseased or morbid structures found in the tissues and organs within the thorax, abdomen, and brain case. It wasn't until the second edition of 1797 that he added the briefest of symptoms to the descriptions of morbid anatomy. How to read anew what was found? What did he make of the tubercle, freed from the constraints of individual patient histories?

Morbid Anatomy was well stocked with observations of tubercles: in the lungs, liver, gall bladder, spleen, and uterus. Baillie declared there was 'no morbid appearance so common' but he used 'tubercle' in the usual general way to refer to growths, swellings, and tumours, so these were not necessarily what we would think of as tuberculous: some were, but not all.[6] Much greater precision came with the addition of the descriptor 'scrofulous'. Scrofulous tubercles (or tumours or swellings, he used all these terms) were more widespread than tubercles per se and had more precise parameters. In particular, he provided a well-defined picture of their contents: 'a white, soft, cheesy matter, mixed with a thick pus', which he decisively informed his readers 'is the most decided mark of a scrofulous affection' wherever this might appear in the body. His list included the pharynx, peritoneum, mesenteric glands, kidneys, renal capsule, testicles, and meninges.[7] This focus on a specific morbid appearance brought to light scrofulous disease in new places: 'I once had an opportunity of seeing two or three scrofulous tumours, growing within the cavity of the pericardium [membrane enclosing the heart]...They consisted of a white soft matter, somewhat resembling curd, or new cheese...a very unusual part of the body to be attacked.'[8]

What about the lungs? Like his predecessors, Baillie found evidence of inflammation, abscesses, cysts, too much water, too much air, problems with the air sacs, the substance of the lungs rendered liver-like, bony, or earth-like in parts. Crucially though, he reported on the extreme regularity with which tubercles were found here, there was, he said, 'no morbid appearance so common'. Many might have agreed with that, but his precision in delineating their precise location was new and he threw light on the gland issue that had troubled Morgagni. The 'rounded, firm, white bodies' were fashioned in the tissue holding together the air sacs. They were not invisible glandular tissue made large: 'There is no glandular structure in the cellular-connecting membrane of the lungs'.[9] Initially no larger than the head of a pin, the tubercles clustered, growing together to produce larger pathologies, typically the size of a garden pea, though subject to 'much variety' of extent. He reported on how larger, tuberculated masses developed from their smaller brethren containing the 'thick and curdy' scrofulous pus. Abscesses followed the suppuration of these masses: when the pus was in great abundance it came to resemble the pus of a common sore. Sound or damaged lung tissue separated the smaller tubercles or larger cavities. Sometimes upon opening tuberculated lungs it appeared that the majority of the tissue had been transformed into 'a whitish soft matter, somewhat intermediate between a solid and a fluid, like a scrofulous gland just beginning to suppurate'. Such pathology he attributed to deposition of the 'scrofulous matter' in the tissue of the lung without being bound by the tubercle's coat. The progression of tubercle to abscess was manifest in the patient as 'Phthisis Pulmonalis [pulmonary consumption or phthisis]; one of the most destructive diseases in this island'.[10]

Reading Baillie's wonderfully clear text, the modernist would urge him to join up the scrofulous matter strewn throughout the body, like a series of dots, and then stand back and realize that this was all the same: the same pathology means the same disease, wherever it is found. He seemed so tantalizingly close to making that connection. He didn't. René Laennec did.

'The True Anatomical Characteristic'

René Laennec (1781–1826) has often been portrayed as new: champion of the new concept of specific lesions for each disease; part of the new way of examining the body; part of the new domination of the doctor over the patient. For the tubercle, his was the new mantra that this lesion must be present in cases of phthisis—'the true anatomical characteristic'—if it wasn't, the disease was by definition something else.[11] And he invented a new piece of diagnostic equipment—the stethoscope—the better to listen to the consumptive chest and announce the presence of his 'unit lesion'.[12]

Laennec was also old (neither new nor old should be read as judgements). Amid the materialism of revolutionary France he retained a belief in a life force—a belief that the phenomena of life are due to an immaterial force—which he set alongside the other components of the body, the solids (organs) and liquids. His MD thesis (1804) reconciled various Hippocratic passages with contemporary ideas. A royalist and Catholic, his career was initially hampered by a conscious conservatism, which sat awkwardly alongside the avowed atheism and republicanism of post-revolutionary France.

It was an exciting and exacting time to be a medical student. Laennec counted the great names of Paris medicine among his teachers and fellow students. He benefited from an education uniting medical and surgical knowledge (the better to produce doctors for Napoleon's military campaigns, and attempt to meet the needs of the French population). He learned the new anatomo-clinical methods, relating findings at post-mortem to the symptoms observed during life and the keeping of careful numerical records. A skilled dissector, Laennec taught his skill to fellow students to help support his education, and published papers on pathological anatomy. Unable to obtain an official position, he established a lucrative practice among the clergy, returning émigrés, and Bretons living in Paris (Laennec was born in Quimper, Brittany), worked for a medical charity, and continued his investigations into the pathological results and physiological processes of disease in the body including phthisis. He probably also suffered from it himself.

Things changed for the better with Louis XVIII's return to the French throne in 1815. Laennec's loyalty was rewarded with an appointment at the Necker Hospital in September 1816. If private practice provided circumscribed research material, he was now empowered by the sheer volume of patients and the 'clinical contract'.[13] The hospitalized, treated free of charge on the wards, provided teaching and research material. This continued after death, at autopsy. Most of the thousand-plus patients admitted annually to the 100-bed Necker Hospital during Laennec's tenure (1816–19, 1821–3) were in end-stage disease. Chronic symptoms of the heart and lungs were common. Laennec examined his patients according to the four pillars of French hospital medicine: inspection (looking), palpation (feeling), percussion (tapping), and auscultation (listening). He augmented listening through his discovery of 'mediate auscultation', using an instrument or mediator: the stethoscope. What started out as a rolled tube of paper in 1816—the better to hear the chest sounds of a plump female patient—quickly became a machined wooden tube. With the stethoscope, a trained ear, and a prepared mind, Laennec was able to precisely appreciate in the living patient the lesions previously knowable only after death.

Laennec began his career in stethoscopy with diseases of the heart. In sorting out those different pathologies he was obliged to work against the background clamour of normal and abnormal breath sounds. They soon moved to the foreground. In the summer of 1817 he coined the term 'pectoriloquy' (literally 'the chest speaks') for the sound of the patient's voice, heard not from the mouth but through the chest wall. Moving the stethoscope carefully over the entire chest, front, and back, it was possible to hear a modulation in the volume of the transmitted voice, which 'seemed to come directly from the chest and pass completely through the central canal of the cylinder'.[14] Where the sound increased, the lung had cavitied. A cavity meant phthisis. He soon discovered, and other stethoscopists pointed out, that it was not quite such a neat fit. By December 1817 Laennec acknowledged that dilation of the large airways— bronchiectasis (from which George Orwell suffered along with pulmonary tuberculosis)—resulted in a very similar sound.

This was 'broncophony' ('voice of the airways'), not pectorilo-quy. However, such subtleties were grist to the mill: the ear could be taught to differentiate between them.

Refined listening and its new language delineated specific conditions by lesion, allowing their earlier detection, ultimately before patients considered themselves to be sick. It reduced patients' input to the medical encounter. Their role was now less to describe their symptoms and more to passively acquiesce with the demands of the doctor during a physical examination: 'Breathe in, breathe out; cough please and again please.' It wasn't infallible and it required considerable skill and practice, but what potential!

While still a student, and long before he invented the stetho-scope, Laennec argued that there was only one form of phthisis and it always involved tubercles. He employed a complex typology of their different forms and developmental patterns, depending on where they appeared in the body, their structure, and their contents. So much he might be said to share with oth-ers, especially his colleague G. L. Bayle (1774–1821), but Laennec gradually struck out on his own. He simplified his typology. In 1812 his tubercles were reconceptualized as one of four kinds of growth or 'accidental tissue', which were 'non-analogous'—they differed from any of the body's normal tissues. After his direct experiences at the Necker, much thought, and discussion with colleagues (some friendly, others less so), he subsequently issued his manifesto on the singularity of tubercles as part of his *Treatise on Mediate Auscultation* (1819). It's worth dwelling on.

Laennec described how tubercles first appeared in the lung in their 'miliary' form: 'small semitransparent grains, greyish or colourless', ranging in size from a millet to a hemp seed. From the miliary developed the 'crude or immature' tubercles. These were either larger individual lesions, 'yellowish and opaque, at first in the centre', then 'successively throughout their whole substance' or fusions of several tubercles creating 'larger masses' of the same colour and with the consistency of 'very firm cheese'. At this stage the otherwise healthy tissue between the tubercles began to be compromised, growing 'hard, greyish, and semi-transparent...by means of a fresh production and seeming infiltration of tuberculous matter, in its first or transparent stage, into the pulmonary tissue'. Alternatively such changes in the lung tissue could occur without the tubercles being initially visible, but then 'yellow opaque points' appeared and converged to 'convert the whole diseased space into a tuberculous mass' of the crude or immature kind.

'After a very uncertain period' these crude tubercles 'softened, and finally liquefied' from their centre outwards. The tuberculous matter so produced was of two kinds. Either thick pus, a deeper yellow than before but without any smell, or a curd and whey mixture part opaque cheesy material, part thin, colourless (unless blood-stained), transparent liquid. Reaching a bronchial tube on its destructive path, the matter could then find its way out of the body after a bout of coughing. Laennec warned that it was rare indeed to find only one of these cavities. The usual pattern was an encircling of tubercles variously softening and discharging their load of tuberculous matter into the established cavity so that over time the 'continuous excavations so frequently observable...sometimes extend from one extremity of the lungs to the next'. Thus could the chest 'speak', he said.

He described how the blood vessels and bronchial tubes were moved aside by the growth of the tubercle. He detailed various membranes including a cartilaginous lining, making a continuous surface between the interior of the cavity and the bronchial tube into which it emptied. He reviewed a few anomalous developmental patterns, but insisted these were 'mere varieties', not distinct lesions. As such it was an all-inclusive survey of the development of the tubercle lesions in the lung in phthisis. It wasn't just a thorough report listing what kinds of pathological changes were found in the region of the body, on a particular organ or tissue; Baillie had been pretty good on that. This was a conscious emphasis on the physiological processes in and progress of a specific disease. It happened in essentially the same way in anyone. Laennec was not finished yet. For it was not just in the lung that tubercles followed such a pattern: this was his master-stroke.

'In consumptive patients it is very uncommon to find the tubercles confined to the lungs…There is perhaps no organ free from the attack of tubercles, and wherein do we not, occasionally, discover them in our examination of phthisical subjects.'[15] Of course you had to understand what you are looking at, and Laennec chastened his predecessors (Bayle in particular) for missing the 'grey semi-transparent character of them in their earlier stage' and for not making the connection between these and the 'yellow opaque tubercles' which they became. Baillie and Bayle both saw them; each read them differently.

Laennec's register of extrapulmonary tubercles makes for depressing reading: a body could be riddled with them. The presence of tubercles would be associated with painful symptoms—'almost always they occupy the intestinal coats, at the same time, and are the cause of the ulceration and consequent diarrhoea so general in this disease'—or be an associated cause of death: on 'the surface of the peritoneum and pleura…they are found small and very numerous, usually in their first stage, and occasion death by dropsy before they can reach the period of maturation'. He explained the collapsed spine by their presence in the 'substance of the vertebrae or the point of union between these and the ligaments'. Pott's disease—a condition of lower-limb paralysis following spinal curvature named after Percivall Pott (1714–88), who delineated its pathology, was in fact a consumptive condition. After the guts, tubercles were found most commonly in the bronchial, mediastinal, cervical, and mesenteric glands and least often in the voluntary muscles. One of his patients, whose neck muscles were compromised by tubercular degeneration, had no pain but difficulty with movement. After death the nearby lymph nodes—whose swelling would likely have been diagnosed by others as the different disease, scrofula, were 'full of tubercles and much enlarged'. The most compromised part of the muscle 'was converted into tuberculous matter, firm and consistent'; the least affected part 'was in its early stage, grey and semi-transparent'. It was the pathology of the lungs all over again.

Laennec had unified a myriad group of pathologies, traced the lesion to the symptoms and given new meaning to 'tubercle'. He didn't propose a cause—that for him was unknowable—nor offer good news about therapeutics. He didn't take the world by storm. Such breakthroughs are rarely that, except with historical hindsight. A far greater continuity predominated among clinicians and their living patients. Tubercles might have made it to the forefront of a consumptive's pathological anatomy and with the aid of the stethoscope, yielded earlier diagnosis, but they were in the background of their subjective experiences.

'They Wait with Impatience'

In the early 18th century, European's most renowned clinician, Herman Boerhaave (1668–1738) of Leiden, received a letter from an apothecary asking for an opinion concerning one of his patients, a 23-year-old merchant. Postal consultations from lesser practitioners or patients were part of an eminent physician's routine. In this case, the apothecary reported that the merchant had fallen 'suddenly into a spitting of blood' in March of the previous year (the letter is undated). This 'throwing up' of 'pure red blood by means of a gentle cough' lasted for three days. The symptoms continued for a while with a spitting 'four times a day' before it 'diminished in quantity', subsequently became mixed with phlegm, and then ceased altogether. A dry cough lingered, but he was eating well, seemed to be recovering, and attended to his work as usual. As the man was slightly built, his friends and family failed to notice that he was beginning to lose weight. When realization struck, he tried taking goat's milk over the summer, but there was little change. In the autumn the cough turned wet. Colds were prevalent, but the merchant's cough dragged on beyond the ordinary course, increasing in frequency and violence over the winter and now accompanied by 'tough viscid *Phlegm* of a green colour'. Then the night-sweats began: the merchant was exhausted and had little interest in food. On the positive side, the apothecary reported that his patient told him he was free from pain in his sides and chest. The stools were 'every way as usual in health', the urine 'pale'.

The apothecary urged an early reply: 'they wait with impatience'.[16] When it came, it contained an unequivocal diagnosis: 'After carefully considering the case, I am of opinion that the patient labours under a real consumption', which began after a 'suppuration'—a festering—in the lungs following the blood-spitting episode. Boerhaave would have been all too familiar with the apothecary's description. Many of his other virtual and real patients shared the merchant's symptoms.

Boerhaave offered a poor prognosis: enfeeblement, wasting, and drenching night-sweats indicated the consumption's advanced course, but all was not lost. He proposed a regimen of exercise, rest, and diet and a course of medication. Like Sydenham, Boerhaave recommended the merchant take to his horse: 'The gentleman should ride as much as he can every day when his stomach is empty, and indeavour [sic] to increase his journey's by degrees.' He was to cultivate a regular sleep pattern—in bed at eight o'clock and rising early. It was essential that the bed was 'well dryed [sic] in a room on one of the high floors'. Boerhaave advised an equal mixture of fresh mead and milk as his 'ordinary drink'. Approved food was more varied: 'all kinds of grains prepared any how, soft herbs and greens, milk, river crabs, shelfish [sic], and now and then...a little fresh flesh'. He should eat little and often, like a kitten. Between rides and meals, at three-hourly intervals, he was to take pills, followed by a liquor and, before retiring to bed, a draught. Boerhaave supplied the prescriptions and suggested the patient 'make a tryal [sic] of what I here propose for two months, to see if it will do any service'.[17]

'I Pray God May Bless It': Treating the Consumptive

The merchant's fate is lost to us, but the suggestions for his treatment reveal much about the practical understanding of consumption and its management. Boerhaave's brief reference to ulceration reminds us of what anatomists found under the skin. Treatment centred on dealing with visible symptoms too: what the patient actually suffered. In the modified model of the early 18th century, the language of the humours referred to their

acidic qualities and emphasized a physicality, literally a sharp-
ness and impeded flow: the result of the new interest in chemistry and physics as applied to the living body. Restoring their
balance was still essential to therapeutics, but the nerves and
the substance of the body would begin to play a much larger
role in explaining health and disease as the century progressed.
Balance was imperative here too. The fibres and nerves were to
be toned or relaxed to allow the all-important humoral flow.

Boerhaave's prescriptions (including the invocation of a
higher power—'I pray God may bless it') contained the familiar
in consumption's pharmacopeia.[18] Many were renowned
pectorals (chest medicines). The pills, liquor, and draught he
suggested contained mixtures of several, primarily herbal,
ingredients. This was polypharmacy at its best, for each
attempted the simultaneous treatment of all the merchant's
symptoms, on several fronts. The agitating and exhausting
cough, which disturbed the stomach and digestion, was to be
soothed (liquorice and Peruvian balsam in the pills). However,
the patient must bring up the noxious matter from the lungs,
so expectorants (veronica, hyssop) featured in the liquor. Conveniently these two herbs acted as tonics and stimulants to
combat the lassitude. Along with lemon balm, all three promoted sweating, helping the body rid itself of excess humours,
through the open pores. Frankincense (pills) and goldenrod
(liquor) were astringents, drying up the ulcers and promoting
healing. Sweet myrrh (pills) was an 'antiphlogistic': it countered
the irritation and inflammation of the ulcerated lungs. Betony
and the ever-useful veronica (both in the liquor) aided the
proper digestion of food by the stomach and the resulting
chyle's subsequent assimilation in the body. Along with goldenrod and fennel (again in the liquor) they also quieted any

flatulence. Sleep was an essential restorative, which the night sweats disturbed. Sitting up with a consumptive patient, onlookers heaved a sigh of relief when the feverish tossing and turning, at its worst between two and four in the morning, finally ceased. A patient's despair at his or her desperate condition often worsened in the night, but this seemingly faded upon wakening and the optimism or *spes phthisica* returned. Bedtime draughts contained more balsam to allay irritation while sweet almond oil, a gentle laxative, prepared the body for rest. Lest this was insufficient to achieve a good sleep, Boerhaave included diacodium: syrup of poppies or opium. Reintroduced to Europe in the 16th century, opium would remain a mainstay in the symptomatic treatment of consumption.

Medication was only one strand of the battle against a consumption. Thus although a drugged sleep could be induced, its regularity and the patient's sleeping arrangements required careful attention. Napping during the day was discouraged. Boerhaave's injunction for a dry bed was underpinned by the belief that dampness was harmful to ulcerated lungs; warmth and dryness were potentially restorative. The same duality applied to diet. Medication might aid the digestive process, but foodstuffs were carefully chosen to reverse emaciation. 'Building up' had to be balanced against the all too frequent accompanying diarrhoea. Some continued to think of milk as a virtual specific. Meat might be best taken boiled or in soup. A robust diet was an important preventive in cases of incipient consumption, especially among children. At the end of the century, the meagre food at girls' boarding schools, in particular, attracted attention for its role in helping to bring on the disease.

Not everyone agreed with horse-riding, sometimes it proved too violent for the compromised body, but exercise remained a mainstay. It stimulated the appetite, encouraged the better distribution of the nutritive juices in the body, 'plumped up the solids', and counteracted the consumptive's tendency to spend long hours shut away, indulging in damaging bookish pursuits, by getting them out into the air.[19] The familiar options—walking, driving out in a carriage—were augmented by the unique physicality of sailing. Although the Scot Ebenezer Gilchrist (bap. 1709–74) spent only four days at sea he revived its ancient precedents and promoted it as a cure for consumptions. A ship was constantly in motion. As she rolled, the muscles of the body were required to continually brace and relax the body, standing, sitting, even during sleep. In the belly the viscera were massaged, in the thorax it pumped the lungs up and down, tending to mechanically remove or dissipate obstructions and tumours by the 'repeated friction and gentle kneading'.[20] If all this talk of a rising and falling stomach leaves you feeling queasy Gilchrist would be pleased: seasickness was not an unwanted hazard, but a positive addition to the sailing cure. Rather than beginning with the usual drug-induced vomit, seasickness provided a natural cleansing to begin the therapy. If the seasickness continued so much the better: the cleansing action was amplified by the additional exercise, which restored the stomach's tone and functionality. In a body thus strengthened, ulcers healed and haemorrhages were stopped or retarded.

Sea voyages benefited the consumptive in other ways. It was often asserted that those who lived on or by the sea were less subject to consumptions. Was this not due to the time they spent in its special air? Humid, dense sea air was charged with a rich load of salts, oils of sulphur and bitumen, arising from its waters. Breathed in, the air delivered a chemical dose directly to the part that needed it most. *Pace* Boerhaave, the humidity kept the lungs naturally moist, counteracting hot inflammations: dry heat might turn the blood putrid. The density of the air made breathing easy, easier than the light air of high mountains, which promoted haemorrhages such was the difficulty of breathing. At sea the air was not still. In its movement this 'elastic fluid' mimicked the motion of the water: constantly undulating and shaking, its potency increased. Passing at speed through this maelstrom was highly beneficial. The chemical load notwithstanding, it was yet another form of exercise as the air pressed against the body, counteracting the enervation of dry, warm, serene land air.

In Gilchrist's experience the benefit of travelling to a different climate—Lisbon, the West Indies—was all in the journey. If a voyage failed it was usually because the patients had waited too long before taking to the sea. In this Gilchrist flew in the face of the advice of others who championed the destination's climate (although his book ran through three editions and a French translation). Contradictions didn't matter; indeed they offered hope. For it was in the nature of consumption's chronic, relapsing nature that at length, when the patient was 'as much tir'd of the physicians, as the physicians were of the disease'; if one therapy from the 18th-century medical market-place failed, move on and try another.[21]

Travelling was writ large across the 18th century. The Grand Tour aimed to finish a young gentleman's education, but a health element could be incorporated. The journey took in various warmer European climates where consumptives were advised to spend their time recuperating in better air and perhaps taking the waters as the neo-Hippocratic revival of air, waters, and places gained in popularity. Sometimes families would travel en masse for the health of one of their number and the diversion afforded to all. The distraction of new sights and sounds, even if the comforts of home had to be sacrificed while on the move, were seen as an important element in the treatment of consumption. Keeping up the spirits, preventing morbid thoughts from taking hold, were vital in those of a melancholy temperament, sunk in a consumptive decline. All over Europe, those who had the resources travelled in search of a cure from one watering hole to the next, perhaps Vichy, Aix-la-Chapelle, Spa, or Baden.

The doctor-novelist Tobias Smollett (1721–71) crossed the English Channel in 1763 with his wife. They were both grieving for the loss of their only daughter and he had long been plagued by the consumptive's panoply of fevers, coughs, spitting blood, loss of strength and body mass, asthma, and painful stitches in his side. He pronounced himself free of the dreaded 'impostume' or abscess in the lungs: there was no purulent matter in what he bought up. The Smolletts waited at Boulogne for the summer's heat to dissipate and here Tobias swam in the cold Atlantic Ocean 'with some advantage' to his health.[22] He was a keen advocate of the newish vogue for cold sea-bathing. He didn't say whether he followed completely the elaborate ritual of plunging in head first, repeating the immersions and then being wrapped and left in wet canvas sheets to induce sweating. The shock of the cold water strengthened the overly relaxed fibres, restoring a healthier tone. The succeeding sweating helped shed peccant humours, the pores being readily opened. It was one of a range of recommended cold and hot, sea and mineral water, therapies for consumptives (and other diseases) providing the constitution was strong enough to benefit from the rigours.

The Boulogne air, however, was to be avoided as it was cold and moist. As the season advanced they headed south to

Montpellier and then along the Mediterranean coast to over-winter in Nice. Smollett took a short sea voyage on the way to Italy, for its health benefits, and toured overland from Florence as far as Rome for the change of climate and the beauty of the ruins, antiquities, and art. At each halt he commented on the healthiness or otherwise of the climate for 'pulmonic disorders', affirming or contradicting each location's reputed benefits. In his own case, where there was no ulceration in the lungs, a sharper climate was permissible; when the malady had pro-gressed a softer climate must be found.

With a progressive medical faculty and arrangements for hospital teaching Montpellier offered expert medical opinion as well as climatic advantages. Overtaken again by 'fever, cough, spitting and lowness of spirits', wasting 'visibly every day', Smollett decided to see what advice he might find locally.[23] He engaged in an epistolary consultation with Dr Fizès, a local doc-tor of high repute. It was not a success. Smollett commented disparagingly on Fizès's abilities as a diagnostician and pre-scriber. He feared for those daily placing themselves under his care. This was the other side of the medical market-place: doc-tors good, bad, and indifferent all offered their advice for a fee, and then there were the out-and-out quacks. As specific loca-tions grew in popularity they attracted patients and doctors to tend to them. Consumptives with large enough purses, beset by their chronic condition, could find no end of ways to dispose of their money while losing what remained of their health.

Smollett returned home in 1765 and continued in wayward health. He paid a repeat visit to Bath. The Romans had been the first to exploit its hot and sulphurous mineral baths, but during the 18th century it became the most famous and fashionable of the English spa resorts. By the mid-1740s fifteen thousand visitors were coming each week, many taking one of the seventeen weekly coaches from London. Others spent part or all of the 'season' there: gaming, playing cards, shopping, attending the assembly rooms, taking the waters, seeing the doctor, and being seen against the backdrop of some of the finest Georgian architecture. Smollett exploited it too and with great effect in his novels, describing in mischievous detail the bathers' antics and the doctors' predatory behaviour.

In public view some endured the pumping—being douched on the head—in the King's Bath. Attendants led (sometimes carried) others into the stinking, scum-covered waters dressed in bathing outfits of yellow canvas (white discoloured immediately). After wallowing and watching (or engaging in) the horseplay in the water, bathers ideally changed into dry clothes or wrapped themselves in sheets to be carried home in sedan chairs and took to their beds to sweat. Such was the press at times that many waited and shivered. When they did go home the chair was wet from the previous occupants. All could drink the noxious waters to prescription, perhaps with a little milk or some medications: anything to mask the taste of 'water that boils eggs'.[24] Consumptives joined the scrofulous, scorbutic, venereal, cancerous, gouty, rheumatic, hypochondriacal, hysterical, and nervous. No wonder that the water was loaded with the 'sweat and dirt and dandruff and the abominable discharges of various kinds, from twenty different diseased bodies, parboiling in the kettle'.[25] The otherwise healthy also bathed as a preventive, cleansing a system ripe with overindulgence: a reminder that working on the body, rather than the disease, was the aim of 18th-century therapeutics. Isolation at least was not an added burden for the 'poor emaciated creatures, with ghostly looks, in the last stage of consumption'.[26]

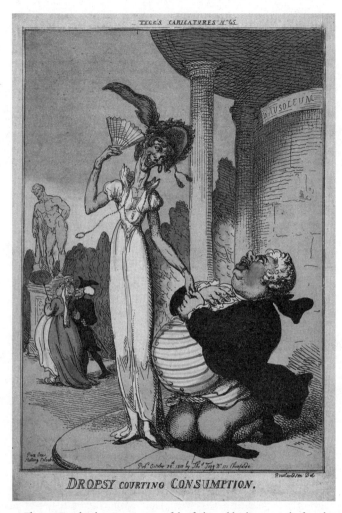

3. Thomas Rowlandson's caricature of the 'fashionable' diseases to be found at the spas: a bloated Dropsy pays court to emaciated Consumption, with a hectic flush to her cheek. (*Wellcome Library, London*)

Smollett has the gouty Matt Bramble, the leading character of *Humphrey Clinker* (1771) move on from Bath in disgust. The consumptive Smollett left too, although he travelled further afield: back to the Mediterranean coast to Leghorn or Livorno in Italy to live. The idea of permanently settling where the air was better was perhaps the logical extension of travelling for health. Find a better place and then settle down. Home was far behind, but the bother of moving on was over. He died in September 1771 ('I am already so dry and emaciated that I may pass for an Egyptian mummy') and was buried in the English Cemetery.[27] The graveyards of Italy contained the mortal remains of visitors and residents for many reasons, but consumption would increasingly be among them.

Too Much of Everything

Had he lived, Smollett might have been interested in the peculiarly English therapy of inhaling gases. In 1799 Thomas Beddoes (1760–1808) opened his philanthropic Pneumatic Institute at Hotwells, a water spa, near Bristol. He hoped to relieve the lot of humankind via the chemistry of factitious or artificial airs. The new gas chemistry had effervesced from the laboratories of Antoine Lavoisier (1753–94), Joseph Priestley (1733–1804) and Joseph Black (1728–99). Beddoes had taught its principles at the University of Oxford. He wondered if excess oxygen in consumptives' blood could cause the characteristic cheeks 'as if painted with a circumscribed spot of pure florid red' and crimsoned lips.[28] After dangerous self-experiments inhaling oxygen resulted in a consumptive-like hectic fever and wasting, Beddoes reasoned breathing oxygen-reduced air would be therapeutic, restoring an appropriate gaseous balance within the body. On a couple of previous occasions he had recommended that his patients lodge in cow houses, to breath bovine oxygen-depleted exhalations, being 'quite persuaded from experience of the power of those fumes to give a healing stimulus to ulcerated lungs'.[29] The production of artificial airs would certainly simplify this and there were plenty of potential patients: hopeless cases were euphemistically referred to as 'Hotwells cases'. Crucially, though, for the radical Beddoes, it could also be offered free to the needy, who were unable to afford to travel for better air. Despite support from England's industrial and Enlightenment elite—Josiah Wedgewood, James Watt (who designed and supplied the chemical apparatus to produce the airs), Davies Giddy, and Erasmus Darwin—the Pneumatic Institute became famous in hindsight not for treating consumption but for bringing a young Humphry Davy and the anaesthetic nitrous oxide or laughing gas to prominence.

However unsuccessful the outcome, Beddoes' motivations are revealing. The number of consumptive patients making up his medical practice and family circle overwhelmed him. Wedgewood and Watt were supportive in part because of the suffering of their children. Brother and sister Gregory (1777–1804) and Jessy Watt (1779–94) were lost to consumption. Beddoes treated the delicate and depressive Tom Wedgwood (1771–1805) with a possible consumption in mind. Beddoes' wife Anna (they married 1794) emerged from the debris of Richard Lovell Edgeworth's consumptive family. Her stepmother and stepsister, both named Honora, had already died from the disease. Her stepbrother Lovell was feared lost, but regained his strength.

For each intimate, there were umpteen faceless consumptives in the surrounding area as Bristol suffered economic and social strain during the 1790s and 1800s. The knock-on effects of the twin revolutions in America and France, disruption of the Atlantic trade routes, and the imposition of taxes to finance the Napoleonic wars pressurized the local economy. At the bottom end of the social scale people simply didn't have enough to eat and the ensuing food riots were violently suppressed. Such straitened living conditions would be likely to accelerate a sufferer's decline from consumption. When and wherever external events united to create misery the same pattern of increased disease and death would ensue.

Earlier in the century, the larger than life George Cheyne (1671–1743) had written on *The English Malady* (1733), concerned about the rising tide of illnesses such as consumptions, hysteria, hypochondria, and the 'vapours'. He believed that the negative effects of overindulgence, relaxing the body's nerves and fibres, lay at the root of all these diseases. Consumption's progress was enhanced where there was a predisposing constitutional taint but it was the ruinous overindulging in alcohol and food—especially meat at the expense of vegetables—that worried him. There was also the hectic pursuit of material goods, which threatened mental destabilization. As the century progressed and England's wealth increased so too did the opportunities for excess. Acknowledged as the consuming centre of the world, England was apparently on the way to becoming the consumptive capital too.

Cheyne's emphasis on body tone and the nerves was part of a wider interest throughout the century. The Swiss Albrecht von Haller (1708–77) studied the body's dual properties of irritability and sensibility. Irritability he defined as muscle's inherent contractibility after stimulation, sensibility as perception by the nerves of external stimuli. The Scot William Cullen (1710–90) devised a nervous basis for all disease. Seeking simplification of Cullen's ideas, John Brown (1735–88) devised a neat dichotomy of asthenic (too little) and sthenic (too much) exciting power within the body. What these theories also had in common was a growing sense that the better classes, compared with their inferiors, had intrinsically more refined nerves, heightened sensibility, greater delicacy, and hence vulnerability to the kinds of nervous sickness that included the consumptions. The poorer classes, with their coarse, insensitive nerves and lack of sensibility, were deemed to be more robust, better able to deal with life's onslaughts, and less likely to fall prey to such disorders: an all too convenient means for the majority to misread their affliction, until it could no longer be ignored.

IV

~oOOo~

CONSUMPTION'S
FASHIONISTAS

I n the 19th century consumption came to be seen in new
ways. It became a fashionable disease, despite the contra-
diction of a painful premature death. Later it would be
remade in a very different way as the new laboratory medicine
finally unlocked its cause. Both were facets of a heightened
visibility.

The image of consumption's refined victims, selected osten-
sibly by virtue of their youth and beauty, endowed it with a bit-
ing tragedy. This disease seemed to single out those 'who have
prepared themselves for the business of life, and whose apparently healthy countenance...seemed to warrant their indulging
in the hope of long and vigorous maturity'.[1]

The consumptive poet or other creative artist crystallized
from its earlier incarnations: 'Sometimes the elegant and cultivated genius shines out with more than usual brightness.'[2]
Female geniuses were doubly at risk, for women in general were
even more subject than men to the fad for a cultivated delicacy,
evident in the ideal of a slim, pale, and interesting beauty. Their
youthful faces were dominated by glittering, overly bright eyes,
while the red spots of a hectically flushed cheek contrasted

delightfully with otherwise alabaster skin. Such a conscious fashion statement was imitated among the trend-setting Romantics who turned away from the age of Enlightenment to bathe in their senses and feelings.

Delicate Males

John Keats (1795–1821) was the youngest of the six great major British Romantic poets: William Blake, William Wordsworth, Samuel Taylor Coleridge, Lord Byron, and Percy Shelley. He was also the first to die. He is sure to be included on any list of consumption's famous male casualties, sometimes depicted as a tragic victim of a dreadful illness, sometimes as the innocent victim of ignorant doctors or vicious critics. Keats's downward trajectory has been written about as a moving, if melodramatic, tale. It is one that typifies the elite male consumptive patient, sets the tone for much of the century, and provides detail on the way consumption was understood and treated in this period.

Keats seemed to embody the long-held association between consumption and genius which he himself interpreted as the necessary balance between human affliction and the production of art in its highest forms: 'Do you not see how necessary a World of Pains and troubles is to school an Intelligence and make it a soul?'[3] The long-standing link between those who shut themselves away and paid too much attention to their books or inner thoughts was updated as the sensibility of the nerves came to the fore. Nerves and fibres were so finely wrought in these individuals that they could easily become overwrought, using up a lifetime's store of energy. Exhausted, they declined thereafter towards a consumptive end. That end was increasingly glamorized, despite the odium of consumption's final throes. 'To cease upon the midnight with no pain' was a fond hope infrequently realized.[4]

Despite his tender years Keats knew this better than some. Before giving himself up to poetry he had studied medicine. A licentiate of the Society of Apothecaries of London in 1816, he then briefly walked the wards at Guy's Hospital as a chosen pupil of the surgical luminary Sir Astley Cooper (1768–1841). It is likely, though, that Keats's first experiences with consumption were familial. His uncle Midgley Jennings (1777–1808) and his mother, Frances (1775–1810), both died of a 'decline' aged 31 and 35 respectively. One might conjecture that these were consumptive 'declines'. The symptoms seem appropriate and the word 'decline' was gaining currency as yet another euphemism for consumption, but there is no certainty. One can be more confident about his beloved younger brother Tom (1799–1818), whom Keats nursed at their home in Hampstead during the final dreadful months.

Tom had been sick for a while, his precarious health necessitating various trips beyond London to prevent the disease advancing and in the hope of some improvement. Early in 1818 Keats joined Tom at Teignmouth in Devon. The southern coastal counties of England were fashionable among the consumptive. Their air and climate received favourable write-ups in popular health manuals. George (the middle brother) was about to marry and emigrate to America. Between rallies, when John and Tom went out on the town, trying to live a normal life, Tom was spitting blood and enduring more serious haemorrhages. The return to London by coach in May became tortuous, the summer and autumn increasingly desperate, and Tom died on 1 December.

In parallel with Tom, Keats also suffered poor health. He had dealt with a self-diagnosed venereal condition in 1817 by taking mercury. After the return from Devon in 1818 he spent some of

June confined to the house with fever. Further febrile episodes and a chronically sore, ulcerated throat cut short a July walking tour of Scotland, forcing an early return in August. The throat and fever continued intermittently during Tom's final illness and into 1819. On 3 February 1819, after a cold journey up to Hampstead from London sitting in the cheap seats on the outside of the stagecoach, he went to bed as soon as he arrived home. His friend Charles Brown heard him 'cough slightly'. Confronted with a drop of blood marking his sheet, Keats announced: 'That is blood from my mouth ... Bring me the candle, Brown; and let me see this blood' ... 'I know the colour of that blood;—it is arterial blood;—I cannot be deceived in that colour;—that drop of blood is my death-warrant;—I must die.'[5] A poet's tendency to melodrama? It was made real later that night when the drop was followed by a haemorrhage.

In little over two years John Keats would be dead. The course of his disease lacked the appalling pace of 'galloping consumption', which often killed in a matter of weeks. It was at the long end of the 'acute phthisis' spectrum. A 'chronic' case could last for several years. But because doctors (and patients) were so reluctant to admit that it was consumption it was often only the final phase of a much longer illness that was regarded as consumption proper. The contemporary assumption was not that Keats had 'caught' his disease from sick family members at some point in the past. Instead the Keatses were understood to share an inherited predisposition. A hereditary tendency could be thwarted but it required a careful regimen and near-constant vigilance. Even then some thought it inevitable that siblings would follow each other to their grave just as children followed parents, grandparents, aunts, and uncles. The less fatalistic warned against courting the kind of ancillary factors that surrounded Keats.

He had foolishly exhausted himself wandering in the Scottish countryside, which while it was a highly attractive landscape for the Romantics, had changeable weather and was often wet and cold. The effects of the unsuitable climate were reinforced when he failed to convalesce properly. After the publication of his long poem *Endymion* in May 1818, several reviews were a shock to the system. Some were harsh and cutting about the quality of the poetry and sniped inaccurately at Keats's supposedly base social origins. In the immediate aftermath of his death some blamed these critics for breaking Keats's literary heart and cited this as a contributing factor in his death. His brother's painful death lowered his already low spirits. Then there were girlfriend troubles. His muse and Hampstead neighbour, Fanny Brawne (1800–65), cast by his friends as '"superficial and vain"…"flirtatious" with "every man she met"' was surely enough to try the resolve of any sensitive young man.[6] Fanny's reputation was later salvaged somewhat but the contemporary perception was that the '"Minx" with a "penchant…for acting stylishly"' had contributed to Keats's heightened mental state and declining bodily strength.[7] Medical opinion firmly supported the notion that 'mental depression operating on a constitution already predisposed to, or labouring under tubercular disease' accelerated 'the evil'.[8] Much of this has little currency today, but in Keats's time such powerful negative effects were deemed important and were publicly discussed—part of consumption's visibility.

Final Throw of the Dice

Keats continued to write and publish poetry (some of the best inspired by Fanny) as his health deteriorated. Indulging in one of the typical consumptive's 'favourite schemes for the promotion of his recovery' he set out for Italy in September 1820 accompanied by his friend, the artist Joseph Severn (1793–1879).[9] He had already abandoned a return to Devon and was forced to acknowledge that the option of serving as a ship's surgeon—a cheap way to gain the prescribed hours at sea and change of air—was hardly realistic. Italy's classical landscape and warmer weather offered a balm to both injured mind and ulcerated lungs, but the journey was a trial. His fellow passengers included other consumptives, one weaker than Keats dying en route. He was at a low ebb when he arrived in Rome in mid-November.

Keats became the patient of James Clark (1788–1870). Eventually Sir James, Clark would become doctor to some of the leading Victorian families, including the Nightingales and the house of Hanover. He would prove a somewhat controversial medical adviser to Queen Victoria, which didn't help his later image. At the age of 30 Clark had accompanied a consumptive patient to the south of France, taking in the Necker Hospital in Paris in 1818 where he learned something of the art of the stethoscope. In Rome he established a practice tending to English expatriates—many of whom were consumptive—and wrote up his experiences as *Medical Notes on Climate, Diseases, Hospitals and Medical Schools in France, Italy, and Switzerland* (1820). Useful tips for Rome included choosing a residence on the Piazza di Spagna. The streets in its vicinity were sheltered and offered the best walks when the weather was fine. Keats had settled at number 26. St Peter's Basilica provided a useful place for exercise. Its constant temperature recommended it as a place to stroll during poor weather while the surroundings provided a much needed distraction for the fretful. For the journey to and fro

Clark cautioned against the use of an open carriage. Long visits to cold museums and churches must be avoided too. In the cold the blood was sent inwards from the extremities to the internal organs, which became congested, increasing the disease there, with deleterious consequences.

Perhaps his most important advice was that where pulmonary consumption had advanced and suppuration taken place in the tubercles in the lungs, the patient ought to stay at home. At this stage 'little or no benefit is to be expected from a change of climate in the cure of disease; and further, that by the great and numerous inconveniences and discomforts of so long a journey, the fatal termination of it is more frequently accelerated than protracted'.[10] As with many of his other patients, this advice came too late for Keats, but Clark was still an obvious choice to be his doctor during Rome's winter invalid season, where the equable climate was rated reasonably highly and there was plenty to do and see, to keep the mind gently active but not overstimulated. Madeira was boring but its relatively constant year-round climate was perhaps the best he advised. Thomas Wakley (1795–1862), founder of *The Lancet*, would see out his last tuberculous days there.

Clinical acumen was probably enough to tell Clark that his patient Keats was near the end. Already a champion of the stethoscope, he particularly stressed its potential for accurate prognosis, the better to avoid raising false hopes. Clark considered incipient pulmonary consumption might be prevented from a fatal course by careful management over a number of years, but he was firm about the attention to detail required to achieve this. Advanced pulmonary consumption remained incurable. It could at best be 'managed' to make the patient somewhat more comfortable.

It is these attempts to assist a dying man that brought Clark his posthumous ignominy. With the benefit of hindsight he has been judged to have precipitated Keats's death more than the harsh critics or Fanny's flightiness. Yet the rationale for Clark's prescription was sound in the context of the time. Following Laennec, he regarded tubercles in the lung as both consumption's 'essential character and immediate cause'. The tubercles were the result of a 'morbid condition of the whole system' because of a hereditary disposition, functional disorders of the basic life process—such as digestion and assimilation of food—or most likely a combination of both.[11] The result of this, what he termed a 'tubercular cachexy', was the prolegomenon to consumption. As the pathology of the tubercles increased there was a corresponding decrease in the capacity of the lung tissue. The chest could not be fully expanded nor could the blood circulate as freely as it was wont. The result—'a plethoric state of the pulmonary system'—was too much blood in too little space. Should the size and type of the diet and the exercise regime both fail to be titrated to meet this impaired state, the lungs would become inflamed, the tubercles tend to suppurate, and the patient haemorrhage. Such inflammation was not restricted to the lungs: it became a general state of the body.

A similar congestion of the mucous membranes in the abdomen, as the blood supply again exceeded what the tissues could tolerate, led to haemorrhaging from the bowels. Should the patient survive these trials he or she would remain at risk of an inflammation elsewhere, so death could follow an apoplexy or the inflammation of some other major organ. Evidence that the body was trying to counteract its plethoric condition and calm an agitated circulation was to be found in the tendency to haemoptysis. The symptomatic remedy therefore was to quieten the system by altering diet, using medication, inducing rest, and perhaps prophylactic bloodletting. In a crisis—a haemorrhage—this might involve letting large amounts of blood.

Called in by Severn in mid-December 1820 after Keats had 'vomited near two cupfuls of blood', Clark immediately let 'about 8 ounces of blood from the Arm: it was black and thick in the extreme'.[12] The next day the same occurred. Clark's instructions were to keep Keats on a low diet—one that would suppress the body and tend to curb the production of blood. Clark's wife helped prepare Keats's diet to her husband's order, but the patient clamoured for more and different food from Severn. Keats was understandably 'weak and gloomy' but giving in to his demands only brought on a 'tormenting Indigestion'.[13] By Severn's account Clark was very caring, but Keats was beyond hope. There were brief interludes when Keats's symptoms subsided but the overall trajectory was downwards. He died in Severn's arms on 23 February 1821. Both men had suffered great distress over the final weeks, even if Severn's kindness to Keats and Keats acting as his muse helped make Severn's name as an artist. Asked if such patients should embark for Rome, Clark was most likely to respond that it would end only with the early filling of another grave in a foreign churchyard marked by a poignant headstone. Such quiet memorials—Keats's contained his own words 'Here lies one whose name was writ in water'—formed potent symbols of consumption's public persona.

Fostering the Lady Consumptive

Happily Keats's love Fanny Brawne continued in rude good health. It was thought, however, that women of her class and better faced particular consumptive dangers from their life-styles. As a fashionable young woman Fanny would have worn the clothing typical of the Romantic age and relatively fortunate social position. Laennec might have been delving into the horrors within the body, but it was to be adorned with the clothes inspired by the rediscovery of ancient Greece and Rome.

Out went the corset, designed to give the body a cylindrical shape and push up the breasts to peep alluringly over its top. In came delicate floating fabrics—muslins, lawn cottons, or batiste—cut in the empire style with its high waist, low neckline, bare shoulders and arms. A potential danger, with only the merest hint of a wrap for additional warmth. Of course there were warmer layers—fashionable pelisses with a military trim and bonnets—but there was still plenty of potential for dangerous chills for the careless, or so the medics warned. Indoors, overheating the rooms could compensate, but beyond the reach of the fire one might step into the cold and experience an immediate chill. Pretty, delicate thin-soled slippers looked lovely, but allowed the cold to creep up. For the possibly consumptive thick-soled shoes, however ugly, must be worn when walking on cold floors.

Excessive exposure to the sun was eschewed for different reasons in the 19th century. A brown skin coarsened by the elements was the mark of the less sensitive, less refined lower classes. White skin, red cheeks, and red lips had been favoured in Europe since the medieval period. It reached new heights of desirability for the Romantics when combined with a wilting demeanour, dangerous slightness of form, and pretended exhaustion—essentially the visible effects of consumption on the body—even among those who were healthy. It was a fine line between an authentic decline and an assumed one. Light clothing, incipient anorexia, and long, idle hours spent indoors would not themselves lead to consumption, but they hardly prepared the body to resist its onslaught. A schedule of cold bathing was a popular preventive regimen, obtainable at health spas. The European leader was Vincenz Priessnitz (1799–1851) whose enterprise at Gräfenberg, Silesia attracted patients and doctors eager to imitate it back home. It reached its most exalted heights in Britain at Malvern in Dr James Gully's (1808–83) hydropathy establishment. Cold-water hydopathy was underpinned by the belief that the body's inability to withstand the effects of being chilled was a leading cause of the inflammation that either gave rise to tubercles or excited these deposits to suppurate. Strengthening to resist the effects of cold by a course of frigid bathing was akin to an inoculation for smallpox.

The cultivation of adult female delicacy began in childhood. Many girls of the upper classes, those living in genteel poverty or sent to be educated at boarding schools, were confined without sufficient exercise in the strengthening fresh air. They spent too long at their lessons; beyond the schoolroom they were engaged in such sedentary occupations as embroidery or other kinds of fancy work and sketching. It was this kind of inactivity that early feminists railed against, not least for its deleterious effects on a girl's health. The novelist Jane Austen has her young women 'walking out' frequently even though the older males protectively counsel staying at home should the weather be inclement.

James Clark believed that a confining lifestyle would lead to a diminished circulation at the surface of the body and extremities. Forced inwards the resulting congestion of the organs of digestion and assimilation would lead to constipation and irritation. (Early involvement of the intestines via the lymph glands, a condition known as *tabes mesenterica*, was indeed more common in childhood because children ingested the then unknown bacillus in their milk.) The visible symptoms were poor skin tone and colour, 'cutaneous eruptions, chilblains, sore glandular swellings and not unfrequently curvature of the spine'.[14] The last might indeed be the crumbling bone in tuber- culosis of the spine (Pott's disease) and raised a more specific alarm call. Some prescribed the use of backboards and other mechanical supporting and straightening devices, worn during long periods of forced immobility. Others advised exactly the opposite: 'Let her be removed to some healthy part of the coun- try, where she can enjoy, free from the injudicious restraints of boarding schools, abundant exercise in the open air, a plain nutritious diet, and, have only moderate mental occupation'.[15] Clark warned against concentrating on restoring the incipient curved spine alone, for strengthening only those muscles would not restore the general health of the body. He referred again to the deleterious conditions in girls' boarding schools, soon to be set before the public in Charlotte Brontë's (1816–55) *Jane Eyre*. Jane's experiences at Lowood were a fictionalized version of Charlotte's own trials at the Clergy Daughters' School at Cowan Bridge, Lancashire which she shared with her two elder sisters Maria (1814–25) and Elizabeth (1815–25), and the younger Emily (1818–48).

Bringing potentially consumptive daughters home from such institutions was insufficient if they were immediately given over to the 'habits of fashionable life', when 'a few months of dissipation often turn the scale'.[16] When sickness hit at Cowan Bridge the Brontë sisters were brought home to Haworth but not for the dubious pleasures of a 'fashionable life'. Maria and Elizabeth died of pulmonary consumption within weeks of their return in May and June 1825. Passing support for the every-day basis for Clark's concerns with the way girls were treated is revealed in an early letter Charlotte wrote to her father report-ing that their brother Branwell had been drawing landscapes from life, while the three girls worked indoors copying other pictures, although walking the hills around the Haworth par-sonage was a favourite pursuit of the Brontë women as young adults.

By the time *Jane Eyre* was published in 1847 the flimsy muslins had given way to the evolving Victorian silhouette: large-shoul-dered, puffy gigot sleeves, and lowered, more defined waists. The corset returned and with it concerns about its deleterious effects on the body. When the passion for large sleeves collapsed mid-century, the corset tightened. It extended downwards over the hips to nip in the waist to the desired waspish dimensions. If the chest could not properly expand respiration was necessarily imperfect: imperfect respiration prevented the proper function-ing of the lungs. Constricted lungs hardly permitted the kind of active physical exercise conducive to general good health and reinforced the persisting fashionable frailty of women.

The Victorians took this to new heights by encouraging their cult of invalidism among those who could afford it. Being sick could be a full-time job: the hysterics and neurasthenics come readily to mind. Invalids of all kinds were supported by a bur-geoning industry of care assistance, helpful technology, and therapeutic retreats of various kinds. If many fancied them-selves sick, far more were and many of these were consumptive. In 1849, when Charlotte Brontë took sister Anne for a 'holiday' to the healing waters of Scarborough, they stopped at York to view the Minster. The dying Anne was too sick to walk, but this difficulty was easily overcome by sending out for a bath chair in which she could be wheeled around. Scarborough was depressingly well set up with plenty of lodgings designed for the sick. Anne died in one of these on 29 May, grateful 'death was come, and come so gently', apparently secure in her belief in universal salvation.[17]

Female consumptives who conducted themselves with dignity during their illness and death were seen as providing valuable examples of religious piety. A French Carmelite nun, Thérèse Martin (1873–97), described her spiritual and physical journey as her consumption progressed in the autobiography *The Story of a Soul* (1898). An inspiration within the Catholic Church, she was canonized in 1925. Tubercular lives and deaths were often recounted by the family members who had sat up and prayed with them through the fevered nights and seem designed in part to comfort the living. Caroline Leakey (1827–81), the author and philanthropist, memorialized her sister Sophia's death in 1858 in an Evangelical magazine. When Caroline died a further sister, Emily, thought it worth reproducing in her biography of Caroline, *Clear Shining Light* (1882). Caroline reported how, after being tempted by the devil in the days leading up to her death, Sophia's faith triumphed and her countenance reflected the spiritual victory and shed its signs of suffering: 'Her face was as it had been the face of an angel.'[18] It was a consciously crafted, potent, and enduring image, which lasted for much of the century. It was also artificial and perhaps reflected the desires of the onlooker rather than the reality of the patient. Sophia's own account more realistically referred to the real world concerns of having the strength only to 'sleep or cough' rather than arrange her features into a beatific readiness for heaven. Already a role for women to play in the privacy of the domestic sphere, the consumptive heroine reached public performance in various forms as the visibility of consumption grew.

Verdi's Violetta

Just as it is easy to spot the consumptive among the 19th century's creative heroes and heroines, a list of their depictions in fiction can be rapidly drawn up. Some were modelled on real victims, blurring the lines between truth and story. Also blurred are the boundaries of social class and the popular tropes of disease as punishment and redemption. Among the most famous females are Francine in Henry Murger's *Scènes de la vie de bohème* (1851) and Marguerite in Alexandre Dumas *fils*'s *La dame aux camellias* (1849). These novels were realized as plays and operas—*La bohème* (1896, 1897) and *La traviata* (1853). Opera as tuberculosis reached an apogee in the 19th century.[19]

Dumas used his lover, the elite courtesan Marie Duplessis (born Alphonsine Rose Plessis, 1824–47), as the basis for Marguerite. Giuseppe Verdi and his librettist, Francesco Maria Piave, renamed her Violetta Valéry in the opera. The Marguerite–Violetta character typifies the notion that the predisposition to consumption was not only hereditary, but could be induced by bad living. She also broadens the visibility of suffering from consumption beyond the artistic and social elite, even if this comes at the price of blaming the victim. While the poor might have little choice about the way they lived and worked they were frequently condemned for it. Those who pursued a bohemian lifestyle of whatever social class similarly brought disease and death upon themselves. A lax moral mentality, irregular hours, and overindulgence in alcohol and sex easily transformed a healthy, beautiful body into one ripe for sickness and destruction. Virtuous men who succumbed to such female temptation were exposed to ruin.

Violetta lives at the extreme—enduring bouts of hectic fever, coughing, and haemoptysis—aware of a life foreshortened. She regards her hedonism as the only cure for the disease she suffers, until Alfredo's redemptive love offers a different solution. The dangerous and debauching city, Paris, is briefly swapped for the purported bucolic health of the countryside. Violetta appears to be in better health. This is an illusion that in the original stage setting was reinforced by the presence of a large fireplace to warm her. She follows Alfredo back to Paris where his father persuades her that she must renounce him for the good of their family name. He cannot see her internal transcendence from courtesan to decent woman through the redemptive power of Alfredo's love. Violetta reluctantly acquiesces and ugly scenes with multiple misunderstandings culminate in Alfredo engaging one of Violetta's escorts in a duel.

Denied respectability through a bourgeois marriage by her past, it seems that only through her death by consumption can Violetta find redemption and the lovers be set free. Her rapidly advancing disease is now admitted and she is given a prognosis of only hours to live at the opening of the final act. The news brings Alfredo back for a reconciliation and the opera heads towards its climax. Throughout Act III, the structure of the music and its orchestration, the libretto, and the directions for Violetta's movements combine to capture the physical decline of a consumptive. At the very end, suddenly imbued with a sense of optimism and health, Violetta is depicted as experiencing the classic false optimism of consumption, the *spes phthisica*. She rises from Alfredo's embrace, believing she has recovered: 'The spasms of pain are ceasing...In me...is born…I am moved by an unaccustomed strength!…Oh!…But I…oh! I'm returning to life! Oh joy!' The phrasing and pauses convey the reality of her compromised lungs.

Her final note—a high B flat—is a moment of great drama. It demands the greatest artistic licence from a body ravaged by this disease. The energy required for this note, the lung expansion, and the likely condition of the larynx in such an advanced case make it tragically unrealistic. The involvement of the larynx was generally an indication of an advanced pulmonary case, although sometimes the voice could be affected before severe lung disease was evident. Hoarseness could progress to complete loss of voice as the ulceration deepened into the vocal cords.

Such a picky medical critique was less of a problem than Violetta's immorality, which bothered some early opera-goers. The opera's subsequent success in the final decades of the 19th century glamorized the female consumptive death and exposed the disease to a growing public scrutiny. While genius and beauty might be the marks of the disease among the middle and upper classes, and offer a spectacle in the case of Violetta, when it affected the masses, consumption became rather more distasteful.

The realities of the sallow complexion, furred tongue, and fetid breath came to the fore. Many came to regard with distrust prematurely aged faces and painfully thin bodies, wracked by ugly coughing. By definition almost everything in the life of the urban poor contradicted the precautions for those of a consumptive disposition or whose relatives fell victim to the disease. The advice was to avoid 'sedentary occupations, especially in confined and obscure places, a residence in large towns and cities, or in low humid and cold situations, unwholesome or improper diet, imperfect clothing, and long continued functional disease of most organs, but more especially and more frequently of the digestive organ. The abuse of strong spirituous or fermented liquors...'.[20] Only the old association between venery and consumption needed to be added to this list.

In the middle third of the 19th century consumption had to compete in the popular imagination with the acute fevers and above all the attention-grabbing epidemics of cholera that tore through the new industrial cities wherever they burgeoned. Yet consumption gained a heightened visibility though poetry, art, literature, and the stage. By the century's end a new leading public enemy had been formulated. This owed much to the discovery of the causative organism of what gradually became known as tuberculosis—the tubercle bacillus.

V

CONSUMPTION BECOMES TUBERCULOSIS

Seeing the Tubercle Bacillus

The transition from consumption to tuberculosis required new methods in microscopy and bacteriology and a new mindset—one prepared to believe that the tubercle—the key lesion—in the lungs, bones, glands, or wherever, was the result of infection with a micro-organism. As this realization took hold, what had been an unrelated family of disorders was recast as a single infectious disease. It changed the way in which its sufferers were viewed and treated. Tuberculosis, rather than consumption, was now set to become visible in new ways.

In 1882 the German bacteriologist Robert Koch (1843–1910) announced the conclusions of his determined scrutiny of consumption. He had identified its cause, rendered it visible using new laboratory methods, and established that it spread from one person to the next as an infection. For Koch this was nothing less than a new, indisputable understanding of this august disease. The cause of so much suffering and death turned out to be single-celled living organisms, tiny rod-shaped tubercle bacilli. 'Seeing' the bacillus relied upon being able to use a microscope and having an adequately stained sample under the lens. Understanding what to look for, how to pick out the bacilli from the other bits and pieces on the slide, were new skills that could be learned. Others had taught Koch. He honed his bacteriological techniques, on anthrax and the bacteria of septic infections, before tackling consumption. He championed a series of procedures, which came to bear the eponymous name of Koch's postulates to show that the bacilli he had discovered were not just present, but the essential and only cause of the disease.

Koch's earlier work had resulted in a crucial cognitive shift. He believed, and was confident he could demonstrate, how specific living micro-organisms were responsible for specific diseases. Based on experimental observations made in the controlled environment of the laboratory, it was obvious to Koch and his immediate circle that the complexities of consumption were a thing of the past; it had been redefined as the presence in the body of its causal germ. Koch would even bequeath the disease a new name as 'TB'—the abbreviation of *Tubercle bacillus*—gradually entered the medical vocabulary. In 1839 the German J. L. Schönlein had introduced the name 'tuberculosis' during his pathological research to refer to conditions characterized by the formation of tubercles but it had been little used. 'TB' and 'tuberculosis' were the names of the future.

Koch's germ aetiology, and with it the reunification of the tuberculous family of related conditions, were both part of complex debates about diseases, their causes, and their mode of spread. Koch may have been supremely confident but it took time and negotiation for others to accept the facts and their implications. Koch's ideas competed with a range of other ideas. René Laennec had drawn together the pathology of the tuberculous afflictions with his unifying concept of the tubercle. He did not pursue the tubercle's ultimate cause; seeking after it brought only fool's gold. Disease arose from within and often spontaneously, with external factors acting only as an exciting cause on a body in some way predisposed, what was termed the tubercular 'diathesis' or 'dyscrasia'. Laennec's diagnostic acumen and his stethoscope found many followers in Europe and North America but there were challenges to his unitary theory of the tubercular diseases. His fierce rival, François-Joseph-Victor Broussais (1772–1838), continued to pour scorn on the primacy and centrality of the tubercle and on the notion of localized disease. Broussais championed the general inflammation of the tissues, especially the gastric tissues, as the basis for all disease. He explained to his own satisfaction how the tubercle was not the specific and primary lesion in consumption but a secondary manifestation, which could occur in any inflamed tissue. He revised the rationale for the familiar range of quietening, depletive, or anti-phlogistic therapeutic interventions. Many clinicians pragmatically preferred to offer the usual therapies along with the 'opium and lies' so many of their consumptive patients required. Laennec's localized pathology had not yielded any useful therapeutic alternatives and he said himself: 'the cure of phthisis by nature is possible, but not by art'.[1]

The 'British School' were not keen on the centrality and unity of the tubercle. They tended to accept the fundamental character of the inflammatory process, but avoided excessive theorizing about why this might be so. Important here was what the pathologist could see and what the patient experienced. Thus pulmonary consumption was split into a series of symptom-driven 'types'—acute, scrofulous, tuberculopneumonic, catarrhal, fibroid, haemorrhagic, laryngeal, and chronic. According to the leading British authority on the pathology of consumption, Thomas H. Green, the different types resulted from the 'intensity' of the inflammation, itself the product of the 'severity of the injury and susceptibility of the tissue injured'.[2]

In Germany perhaps the greatest patho-physiologist of the mid-19th century, Rudolph Virchow (1821–1902), also rejected a unitary reading of the tubercle. He worked in the laboratory as well as the hospital ward and dead house. He moved beyond the tissues, advocating instead the primacy of the cell. These fundamental building blocks of plants and animals had been discovered as part of the new microscopy of the 1830s. Virchow was at the forefront of cellular pathology and physiology, making a number of basic assertions about the role of the cell in health and disease. All cells came from other cells, he said, and illness was nothing more than the malfunctioning of normal cellular functions. In his view of the pathological process there were no new and distinctive disease cells formed. Contra Laennec, tubercles were not a new kind of tissue produced as diseased tissue was broken down or consumed. Microscopic investigation of tubercles seemed to indicate that there was too much variety in these lesions to regard them all as the same thing with the same cause. Virchow and his followers—the 'German School'—thus rejected the Laennecian specificity of tubercles and the attendant unity of the tubercular diseases.

Consumption as Contagion

To the end of his long and powerful life Virchow also resisted the idea that disease could be caused by something from outside entering the body to wreak havoc from within. The idea of disease-causing germs, either entering via some kind of contagion or arising spontaneously, has a long history, and it is important to differentiate the diverse earlier ways of thinking from that of Koch and his contemporaries. Although consumption was essentially regarded as a hereditary disorder (exactly what seemed to run in families varied through time and place and was not always clear), there were periodic flirtations with its potential contagiousness.

Among the most famous is the Italian Girolamo Fracastoro's (1478–1553) proposal that seedlike contagia could cause epidemics. He was mostly interested in explaining the new disease of syphilis, which swept through Italy, perhaps brought from the Spanish Americas by returning troops, but he did include consumption among other diseases with a possible 'germ' origin. Fracastoro's 'seeds' were wonderfully varied and therefore able to explain any number of different disease outbreaks. They might be either living entities or chemical in nature, arising from sick bodies or decomposing matter or appearing spontaneously in the air. It was possible for them to spread disease by direct contact between the sick and healthy, indirectly by contact with contaminated goods or soiled linens and clothing or some other kind of remote mechanism. Fracastoro did not see these 'seeds'—his was a theory. With the use of the early microscopes in the 17th century the world of the very small was found to include worms and other minute bodies. Their constant association with disease, diseased flesh (occurring after surgery or wounding), or rotten meat was not certain, so ascribing them a definite causal role was complicated and hotly contested.

In 1720 Benjamin Marten, placing himself among the 'moderns', announced his repudiation of existing ideas of humoral causation. Instead:

> The *Original* and *Essential Cause*...may possibly be some cer-
> tain Species of Animalcula or wonderfully minute living
> Creatures, that by their peculiar Shape, or disagreeable Parts,
> are inimicable to our Nature, but however capable of subsist-
> ing in our Juices and Vessels, and which being drove to the
> Lungs by the Circulation of the Blood, or else generated there
> from their proper *Ova* or Eggs, with which the Juices may
> abound, or which possibly being carried about by the Air,
> may be immediately convey'd to the Lungs by that we draw
> in, and being there deposited, as in a proper *Nidus* or Nest,
> and being produced into Life, coming to Perfection, or
> increasing in Bigness, may by their Spontaneous Motion, and
> injurious Parts, stimulating, and perhaps wounding or gnaw-
> ing the tender Vessels of the Lungs, cause all the Disor-
> ders...*Phenomena* and deplorable Symptoms of this Disease.[3]

He stopped short of saying that he had seen these organisms.
Again it was a thought experiment rather than a series of carefully conducted observations, and he had nothing new to add to
either the standard means of prevention or therapy.

In the face of such possibilities it sometimes paid to err on
the side of caution. The Italian city-states of Florence and Lucca
had passed (and repealed) laws designed to prevent contact
with the bodies and goods of the consumptive. The Kingdom
of Naples also passed a public health ordinance in 1782 designed
to prevent the spread of consumption that was underwritten
by its supposed contagiousness. The breath of the consumptive or their body odour and anything that had been in contact
with either was suspected of being a medium of contagion. The
law demanded that physicians report consumptive patients
whose lungs were ulcerated. The sick poor were to be hospitalized. Hospital superintendents must segregate these patients,
keeping their linens and utensils apart from those in general

use. The better off could remain at home or in the temporary lodging taken as they overwintered for their health. Once alerted to their presence the authorities would take and burn their personal effects after death. Anyone who resisted would be severely punished, as would those who attempted to buy and sell such goods (or those taken into or used in the hospitals). What could be cleaned was cleaned thoroughly, and what could not would be burned. Plasterwork, doors, and windows in houses where a consumptive had died must be removed, burned, and replaced with new materials. This might seem wonderfully specific, but they were typical solutions to other diseases—especially plague and cholera—that affected Italy's coastal cities. The costs involved certainly led to a lingering negativity in guesthouse owners towards consumptive tenants seeking the warmth of the Mediterranean. The prejudice extended informally beyond the Kingdom of Naples and outlasted the repeal of the law with Italy's unification in 1860. The game of cat and mouse continued as the sick would hide their condition only to be betrayed by their racking cough and told to move on. Local traditions die hard.

On the other side of the world Chinese medical literature frequently referred to various disease states of depletion and exhaustion approximating to western ideas of consumption. *Chuanshi lao*, or 'corpse-transmitted wasting', was a fatal, often familial, disease in which the internal organs of Chinese anatomy all contained wasting worms.[4] These invisible worms were not necessarily worms per se, but various kinds of unpleasant creatures consuming the body from within. After the death of their host they moved on to a new living body. As they moved on, they transformed into increasingly virulent forms. In the close proximity of the family setting they easily took their toll.

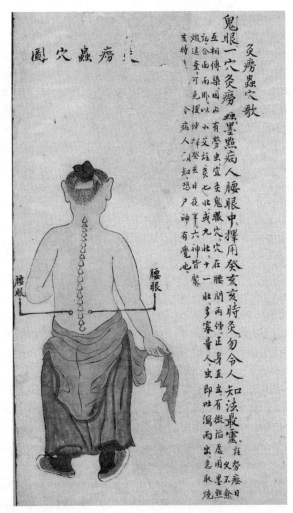

4. Laochong or 'consumption worm' moxibustion chart, in *Record of Sovereign Teachings* (1869). In lingering consumptive diseases a series of moxibustion treatments (burning the herb mugwort), to be repeated seven, nine, or eleven times depending on the patient's condition, at the lumbar eye points (on either side of spine). (*Wellcome Library, London*)

During the 18th and 19th centuries scholars of the 'evidential research' school were cautious about endorsing something they couldn't see and preferred to discuss mechanical causes such as impeded flows of blood and *qi* energies. Nevertheless the worms as agents of contagion remained prominent in popular medical works. When Koch's germ theory reached China these older ideas facilitated its assimilation.

Inoculants, Zymes, and Living Germs

In the mid-1860s the Frenchman Jean Antoine Villemin (1827–92) conducted a series of experiments, taking matter from tubercles and inoculating it into healthy rabbits. Villemin was confident that he had shown the contagiousness of consumption just as glanders could apparently be passed from horses to humans and syphilis from one person to the next during sexual intercourse. Villemin's critics did not deny that localized lesions appeared in the recipient animals but described this as merely 'artificial tuberculosis'. They remained firm in their conviction that, unassisted by the techniques of the laboratory, deep-seated matter from tubercular lesions could not find its way deep inside the body of another person. Where Villemin's work was greeted positively it was seen as an interesting patho-physiological phenomenon, worthy of further investigation. Was it, for instance, analogous with the idea held by some that tubercles could be disseminated within the body as a sort of self-poisoning? Did it not question the views of the 'German School' on the formation of new tissues?

Villemin's ideas stimulated other inoculation experiments. Their successes attracted the attention of those charged with controlling the links between animal and public health.

Although tuberculous matter was not ordinarily contagious, might there be a danger of infection associated with ingesting milk and meat from cattle that showed the same symptoms during life (coughing, loss of weight, general debility) and the same pathology (tubercles) after death? Thus how you practised medicine or used medical knowledge also affected what you made of new research.

In England, William Budd (1811–80) led the charge to full-blown contagiousness and called for consumption to be classed among the 'zymotic' diseases. He cited the throwing off of morbid matter—*materies morbi*—and the patterns of incidence, especially the spread within families to support his case. John Simon (1816–1904), head of the government's Medical Department, toyed with the idea. As consumption and cancer shared a pathology of growths, he wondered if both should be recategorized.

For the majority consumption simply did not appear to behave in the same way as the other miasmatic, zymotic, or contagious diseases, which bedevilled the rapidly urbanizing towns and cities in the 19th century. The generations-long epidemic of tuberculosis had smouldered rather than flared like the classic acute 'fevers' typhoid, typhus, scarlet fever, diphtheria, measles, smallpox, and above all cholera. Each of these had a more perceptible epidemic profile. There was a rich debate on their identity, causation, and mode of spread but after mid-century support grew for the role of 'zymes', hence 'zymotic fevers'. Zymes were thought to be chemicals. The new chemistry of decomposition and fermentation elucidated by another German laboratory scientist, Justus von Liebig (1803–73), offered an explanatory model. Zymes did not in themselves cause disease, but acted as catalysts causing decay within the body. The decay was experienced as the symptoms of disease. Zymes could also be transmitted.

Their role seemed quite plausible but these chemical non-living entities were quite different from the living organisms that fascinated the French chemist Louis Pasteur (1822–95). What began as a study of fermentation—an economically driven inquiry into difficulties facing the French brewing industry—evolved through analogy and experiment into a model of disease causation. He might have begun with silkworms and chickens, but Pasteur and his team moved on almost seamlessly from problems of commerce to threats to human health. Pasteur's endorsement of a living germ theory of disease did not sweep all before it, but reinforced the idea that micro-organisms caused disease. While in hindsight it would be seen as a defining moment in the history of medicine, at the time it served as a stimulus to those already giving up the chemical zymes to investigate the causal role of living germs. Were there different species of germs, each of which caused a specific disease or did they mutate from one form to another and cause different diseases that way? These were the kinds of questions to be answered.

Pasteur's other great triumph was to show definitively (even if he did quietly fudge his experimental results to help out) that these living organisms did not arise *de novo*. There was no spontaneous generation. If wine turned to vinegar, milk soured, a wound became septic, or a healthy person became sick with a specific disease, a micro-organism had landed upon the material or gained entry to the living body. Pasteur's refutation of spontaneous generation reinforced the idea of contagion. Living germs could be passed from person to person directly or if they could survive outside of the body, by contact with some kind of contaminated matter. Understanding how specific micro-organisms continued their life cycle in this way was now to understand anew the symptoms during sickness, the eventual morbid pathological changes, and the way the disease each caused was spread. This was the purpose of Koch's landmark publications.

Making a Laboratory Disease

Koch read his first paper, 'On the aetiology of tuberculosis', at the Berlin Physiological Society on 24 March 1882. The result of a sustained investigation over several years, it was published on 10 April, quickly translated, and disseminated around the world in the medical and general press.[5] Two years later, under the same title, he wrote a more extensive version, giving greater credit to the work of other scientists and showing the development of his ideas and practical research.[6] He described how his project had involved the differentiation and isolation of the rod-shaped *Tubercle bacillus* from a patient's tuberculous matter. In otherwise sterile conditions outside a living body this organism had been gradually coaxed into entering its protracted cycle of reproduction several times over. The resulting colony was declared free from any possible contamination from its original source and large enough to act as a source of experimental material. Koch inoculated these cultured bacilli into healthy guinea pigs, and maintained a second group as a control. When the inoculated animals sickened, they were killed and autopsied. Unlike the controls (which were similarly examined), they had developed tubercles. The same bacillus was isolated once more from the diseased tissue and once more grown in pure culture. The cycle could be continued indefinitely. To Villemin's inoculation procedure Koch believed he had added unequivocal proof of the role of the causal organism. He had fulfilled the experimental protocol he had helped establish as proof of a living germ's role in a disease. At each step it was necessary to adapt existing techniques or design them *de novo* to accommodate the peculiarities of the bacillus. Koch was not short on ego strength, nor did he do it all by himself, but it was an outstanding accomplishment by his laboratory.

In the wake of the first paper, advocates of the *Tubercle bacillus* within and beyond Germany staged demonstrations at medical meetings to reinforce the message, but there was not much doubt that the bacillus existed. Despite Koch's confidence, what required negotiating was the role it played. Was its presence absolutely necessary, just an accompaniment to the disease, or indeed a sequelae of consumption? If there was a causal role how could this be integrated into existing etiological and pathological models of consumption?

A spectrum of opinion emerged. The arch exponents of the germ were at one end. For the ultra-bacteriologists, led by Koch, the 'soil'—the state of the body into which the germ was introduced—was irrelevant. He concentrated only on the bacillus. The human hosts represented nothing more than the series of identical test-tubes in which he had eventually grown his bacteria. Absence of bacteria was equated with health; the idea that they could be present in the healthy was not entertained. At the other end of the spectrum was a small and ever-dwindling group who denied the bacillus any involvement whatsoever. In between were those who joined the new bacteriology with heredity and other established predisposing causes.

For the supporters of this 'seed and soil' middle ground two things were needed to produce disease: 'the presence of the

Tubercle bacillus, and some abnormal state of the pulmonary tissue'.[7] The underlying condition of the body was still an essential component of the disease process. The individuality of the patient retained its significance. Doctors adjusted the reasons why they continued to prescribe the same therapies. Adherents of the inflammatory school, for instance, could interpret the bacillus as the crucial or a common irritant depending on their position on the spectrum. Construed in this way, the new germ aetiology melded into existing constructions of the disease and familiar therapies. Counter-irritants such as mustard plasters were still to be applied. The young Russian-born painter, Marie Bashkirtseff (1858–84), pretty doyen of Parisian artistic circles, rejected this remedy in 1882 for reasons of vanity:

> a blister, that means a yellow stain for a year. I shall have to wear a bunch of flowers, which I will place so as to conceal it for the soirées, on the right collarbone. I shall wait for eight days longer. If the complication which has arisen persists, I shall, perhaps, make up my mind to undergo this infamy.[8]

In September 1883, thirteen months before she died and eighteen months since Koch's discovery, she gave in to her doctor's recommendation: 'I am thoroughly ill. I put an enormous blister on my chest. After that, doubt, if you can my courage and my wish to live.'[9]

The rationale for travel was also easily reconfigured. The more constant, warmer climate of the Mediterranean was now good because the inhalation of cold air irritated bacilli-infected lungs, rather than just ulcerated lungs. Similarly the newer fad for pure mountain air in the European Alps or the American Adirondacks was recast. These elevated locations had a lower bacteria count: fewer bacteria meant less irritation. Reduced

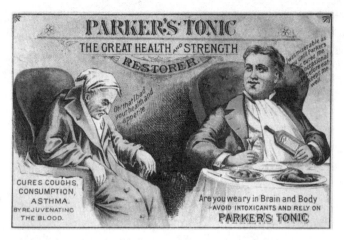

5. An 1870s trade card promises that Parker's Tonic will cure consumption by 'rejuvenating the blood'. The 41.6% alcohol it contained might afford a temporary release, but otherwise this and many other popular 'cures' merely raised false hopes. (*Wellcome Library, London*)

irritation was especially useful in early or inactive cases. Patients could gain the maximum additional benefit from improved lung capacity and stimulation of the pulmonary circulation that occurred at higher altitudes. At the level of the elite, independent patients such as Marie, with her advanced case, the impact of Koch's bacteriology could only be a measured one. For the moment it remained a family tragedy to be dealt with inside the family circle.

Remaking the Social as a Bacteriological Disease

When it came to the tubercular masses things were rather different. In the new Kochian world-view the corollary of a bacterial aetiology was the contagiousness of the disease. As the infectious nature of consumption became accepted, the disease was reconceptualized as a public health problem. The personal stories of the sick poor were reworked en masse as a series of public health emergencies, demanding attention at the national level. Consumption regularly topped the statistical registers of mortality (where these were maintained). It was increasingly seen as a measure of degradation in social surveys. Now it was recast as a contagious epidemic: slow-burning certainly, but real. Its scope was breathtaking—Koch spoke in 1882 of '1/7 of all humans dying from tuberculosis'. If this bald figure requires refinement by today's historical demographers, it serves to remind us what Koch's generation thought they were facing.

Even in England, where the worst of the epidemic was over, the statistics are still sobering. From 1851 to 1910 there were some four million deaths in England and Wales ascribed to tuberculosis (up to 80 per cent of which was pulmonary). This was 13 per cent of the total mortality during these years.[10] Continuing as it had always done to systematically strike young adults, it killed more than a third of those aged 15 to 34 and half of the 20 to 24 age group. Men and women fared differently to some extent, reflecting differences in working experiences and the effects of pregnancy. At mid-century more women than men died of tuberculosis; by the end of the century the balance had tipped the other way with greater male mortality from the disease during these years. Death rates for many diseases were lower in the countryside than in the towns. Consumption was no exception. Rural rates could be inflated by an outflow of the sick that chose or were forced to return home to die, but meagre wages and impecunious living conditions exacted their own levy. Overall though, the trend in England was downward: 3.58 deaths per 1,000 living in 1838, 2.05 in 1879, and 1.33 in 1900.[11]

Fewer people suffered and died from this disease as the epidemic wound down but each active case represented a potential source of infection for others.

In various cities during the 1890s—the decade when the realization of Koch's infectious bacilli gathered pace—deaths from tuberculosis per 1,000 living ranged from 4.6 in Moscow, 4.1 in St Petersburg and Budapest, 3.9 in Paris, 3.1 in Brussels, 2.6 in Stockholm, 2.5 in Odessa and New York, and 2.3 in Berlin to 1.3 in London. The differences in death rates were a snapshot of the history of a protracted global epidemic. The lower rates were to be found in the established industrial cities in western Europe and North America. Wherever manufacturing continued to expand here and in the rapidly industrializing cities of eastern Europe, Latin America, Russia, and Japan, the rates were higher as their epidemics gained pace. Tuberculosis thus appeared to spread and wax around the world. It was not so much that the disease moved—strains of the bacteria were common enough everywhere—rather the social conditions, which precipitated an epidemic's upward mortality slope, were replicated. In these circumstances the chance of tuberculosis spreading from person to person increased—exposure levels climbing ever higher—and the generally lowered vitality of urban populations increased its burden. For each clear-cut case, where the main cause of death was unambiguous, the debilitating effect of one disease overlaid upon another paints an even grimmer picture. Consumption interacted with the two main groups of endemic diseases affecting young urban adults, respiratory diseases (bronchitis, pneumonia, influenza), and gastrointestinal infections. Along with smallpox and measles these left their surviving victims liable to the reactivation of an earlier episode of tuberculosis or could carry off the already debilitated tuberculous.

Low wages and poor working conditions both fostered tuberculosis. In the 1860s Karl Marx and Friedrich Engels grimly commented, 'consumption and other lung diseases among the working people are necessary conditions to the existence of capital'.[12] At the bottom of the pay scale costermongers, porters, and anyone else employed on a casual basis suffered high levels of the disease. Some spent their entire working life in this way. Others, already suffering from tuberculosis, could slip down the social scale, reduced from the higher wages of a skilled craftsman to lowly day rates or sporadic casual labour. Episodes of ill health could reduce a stable family to poverty when the male breadwinner was unable to work full time and retain his former position. Women's wages were insufficient to support a family and even single women struggled. Laundresses and seamstresses, paid by the piece, suffered from high rates of tuberculosis. Among the better-paid men, tin-and coalminers were at risk because of dust, silicosis, and employment in damp closely confined spaces. Those in the printing trades were highly paid but still counted many tuberculous among their numbers. They too worked in overcrowded environments. Typesetters whose job was sedentary were often able to continue to work— and to spread their germs—while they were sick, each cough a threat to their workmates.

The appalling conditions of the early factories facilitated the development and transmission of tuberculosis. The growth of manufacturing concentrated people together in machine rooms for shifts lasting perhaps twelve hours. In the textile industry the deliberately hot and humid air, filled with tiny, irritating fibres, facilitated the flow of the thread and the spread of bacteria. The dust of the potteries and glass-making, and the sharp irritants in metalworking shops were associated with high rates of lung disease. Bakeries might seem more innocuous but in Argentina kneading for long hours through the night in poorly ventilated, flour-dust-filled rooms, hot from the bread ovens, apparently led to high levels of disease among these workers. With such high levels of exposure and the demands of most forms of employment, it would probably be easier to list the occupations that didn't contribute to the incidence of tuberculosis.

In Britain a series of Factory Acts over the course of the 19th century limited the hours worked, improved the conditions within the factory buildings, and made inspections mandatory. Similarly, periodic local and national public health and 'health of towns' legislation slowly cleaned up the cities, dealing with sewage and the deposits of the thousands of animals that provided transportation and food in urban areas. Water became cleaner and more plentiful. Overcrowded, ill-ventilated, ill-lit slum housing conditions were ameliorated in the wake of public outcries usually associated with outbreaks of disease. Vaccination against smallpox was made compulsory, reducing the burden of this disease. None of these measures were directed at tuberculosis, but their slow knock-on effect on the overall health of the working population impacted positively on death rates from this and other diseases. Air quality in towns remained poor. People cooked and heated their homes with coal. The resulting smogs were particularly bad for respiratory diseases. Rising wages meant more spending power, but what to spend it on? Better, more plentiful food perhaps. Food comprised the largest single item in working-class budgets. Imports of tinned and then frozen meat, butter, and margarine increased substantially from the 1870s but an improved diet alone would not turn the tide and there were other ways to spend money.

Many families chose to increase the amount of space in which they lived.

Life remained precarious. Locally, periods of intense poverty or social dislocation caused spikes in consumptive death rates. Overall the death rate from consumption fell over the ten-year period 1861–70 in Salford, a district of Manchester in north-west England. Yet, during the 'Cotton Famine' years, when the American Civil War disrupted cotton imports from the Confederate South and production in the city's mills was severely hampered, tuberculosis death rates in Salford rose against the trend during 1864–7. In straitened circumstances people cut back on the necessities of life. They saved on food—women and children typically going without to keep the breadwinner's strength up—and rent, moving into smaller and hence more congested housing with poorer facilities in less salubrious areas.

If such structural social evils helped fashion consumption as a social disease of the working classes, their rapid amelioration was not the target of immediate efforts to control consumption in the years after Koch's discoveries. Nor would this have been seen as terribly practical given the growing sense of urgency, among the well-intentioned as well as the self-interested. The worried middle classes, sensing both the burden the diseased posed in economic terms and the risk of infection they represented, tended to concentrate on short-term measures to curb the threat. Unsurprisingly then these were often extensions of existing measures of limited institutional facilities, public education, and attempts to change the deviant germ-spreading behaviour of the masses. To the old familiar charges of fecklessness, alcoholism, and venery were added some more specifically dangerous habits. There was a growing pressure to make tuberculosis a notifiable disease the better to corral patients and follow up on their contacts. A burgeoning assortment of local, later national, anti-tuberculosis associations coordinated much of this activity. Internationally a series of tuberculosis congresses reinforced the growing interest in understanding and combating the disease.

At the Dispensary

In 1887 the Scot Robert Philip (1857–1939) opened the Victoria Dispensary for Consumption and Diseases of the Chest in Edinburgh's 'old town'—the first dedicated dispensary for tuberculosis patients. Three rooms in a flat at 13 Bank Street among the crowded tenements of the city was a small beginning, but Philip was convinced of its benefit. On a postgraduate study tour in Europe in 1882 Philip found himself in Vienna just after Koch announced his discovery of the bacillus. Although he had travelled overseas to pursue embryology and gynaecology, he took the opportunity of observing the new bacteriology. Inspired by what he had seen, Philip continued his new interest when he returned home. Over a couple of years he conducted a series of experiments on the effects of the toxic waste products of the *Tubercle bacillus*, which he wrote up in his MD thesis 'A Study in Phthisis'. He obtained the tuberculous sputum for his research from patients attending the New Town Dispensary where he had worked as assistant physician since 1885.

Philip's rationale for a dedicated dispensary was based on this wider dispensary experience, where a dispiriting pattern emerged among the patients. Consumptives would attend the general dispensary for a variable period of time, depending on how long the acute symptoms lasted, and how much faith they placed in the treatment or the doctor. At best they were likely to receive cough mixture, probably containing opiates to suppress the cough. When they became too ill to continue coming to the dispensary they were consigned to the ranks of the chronic or troublesome patients. The main focus of these dispensaries—as was the case with in-patients in the charitable hospitals, which offered care to the deserving poor—was the treatment of acute illnesses. The chronic cases that remained on the dispensary's books could expect an occasional visit at home from an ever-changing rota of medical students; perhaps with more cough medicine. Philip considered consumption an infectious, systemic disease, one that required a thorough approach to both its therapy and attempts to prevent its spread.

His six-point plan for the management of dispensary patients relied upon a comprehensive medical examination on the patient's first presentation and an assessment of their social position. An accurate record of this and all further visits was essential. Patients were to be told how to look after themselves, how to remodel their behaviour to produce careful rather than careless consumptives, so that they become fully aware of the potential threat they presented. Whether this empowered patients to virtuous self-help, or was merely the issuing of draconian instructions, which blamed the victim for their own misfortune, presumably depended upon the tact of the dispensary staff. Patients were to be issued with some assistance in achieving the new hygienic principles by which they must live: 'necessary medicine, disinfectants and sputum bottles, and, where the family circumstances warrant it, of foodstuffs and the like'—hence the social survey.[13] Philip was aware that impoverishment frequently attended consumption and that the dispensary could act as a conduit between distressed families and sources of public or charitable help.

Treating the symptoms was all very well, but Philip stressed that consumptives needed to be 'built up' to help them resist the disease. To ensure patients were containing their sputum in dedicated disinfectant-laden containers, using separate utensils, and cleaning the home and laundry to the required germ-free standards, dispensary staff would visit their homes. This became more critical where patients were house or bed-bound. It also allowed the transmission risks to be gauged. Both in the dispensary and during home visits, patients should be assessed for other treatment options, hospital visits, sanatoria stays, or a transfer to a home for the incurable to die. As with the issuing of additional food, these decisions were informed by medical need and social circumstances. The dispensary was also there for patients sent home from hospital. In a period before many had a permanent relationship with a general practitioner the dispensary sought to ensure continuity of care. Such continuity was important in the moral dimension of consumptive treatment: patients were reminded that they had a duty to get well and to prevent the spread of the germs they harboured. Crucially the dispensary provided an open public information service for consumptives, families, and friends, indeed anyone who wished to know how to deal with and to try to prevent this disease.

Such education of the public was widespread wherever there were concerns about the death rate from consumption. The French had come later than their neighbours across the Channel and the Rhine to realize that this disease was the major killer of the *belle époque*, partly due to poor statistical accounting and partly to various subterfuges designed to avoid ostracism. Once the situation was acknowledged, they were galvanized to educate their citizens, among other measures. Their 'War on

Tuberculosis' included great attention to spitting. The French racked up their antagonism to the once socially acceptable practice. In 1886 the Conseil d'Hygiène et de Salubrité voted to outlaw spitting on the floor in public, calling for the use of spittoons containing sawdust. The sawdust was to be burned and the spittoon scalded with boiling water. In light of the germ theory, the strong class-based social repugnance was now overlaid with fear of disease transmission. When people spat, globs of saliva, liberally dosed with bacilli, landed on the floor, or any other surface. According to the prevailing ideas, once the saliva dried the still potent bacilli would be distributed into the air, floating on particles of dust as the floors were swept. Inhaled into a clean pair of lungs, the disease spread from the sick to the healthy.

It was bad enough that people infected their own space, spreading disease among their family members, but it was perhaps even more important to police public areas. In the workplace for instance, 'A single sick worker can contaminate an incalculable number of his comrades, the foreman, and even his bosses; since bacillus laden crachats [sputum] are lying on the ground everywhere!'[14] Corrective education in communal settings could be carried home. Those who used a handkerchief to catch the coughed up sputum were to be commended but the handkerchiefs had to be carefully dealt with afterwards—without proper care the contents could still act as foci of infection as they dried. The ideal repository remained the spittoon. Its contents required diligent management. Ideally they should be dosed first with a phenol or other preparatory disinfectant and covered. Left open their contents were made available to flies, 'the great traveling salesmen of tuberculosis'.[15] The spittoon

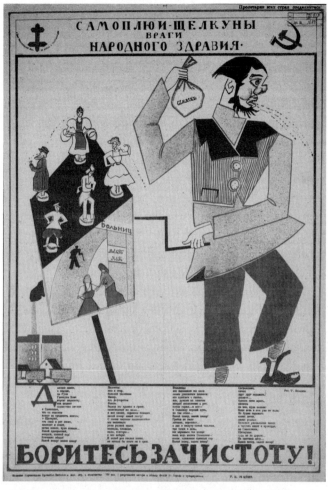

6. Demonizing the tuberculous in 1920s Russia: 'Dirty Vlas', a spitting 'enemy of the people's health'. Education through posters (and exhibitions) was a mainstay of public health campaigns. (*Wellcome Library, London*)

must not be tipped onto dung heaps or garden soil, or chickens pecking for worms might be tubercularized.

Spittle-smeared fingers potentially spread germs with frightening ease. Fears were raised about the contamination of library books; each square centimetre of a printed page housed 43 bacteria, calculated a concerned columnist in *Le matin*.[16] Among the sensible advice was a great deal of hype, even hysteria, which was part of the wider sensationalism around germ aetiologies. It was a boon for the manufacturers of a variety of anti-germ products including 'air-purifying' products such as the Papier d'Arménie sold in France from 1885. Specially prepared blotting paper, soaked in benzoin resin derived from the styrax shrub, released a pleasant odour when burned and purported to cleanse the air of disease-causing germs. It would be more pleasant than the sulphurous acid gas others advocated.

At the Edinburgh dispensary Philip soon added the 'march past' to the regime. The immediate family and contacts of the dispensary patient were strenuously encouraged to submit to a methodical, and perhaps frightening, examination to determine if they too were infected and infectious. Early detection of diseases, the better to deal with them, is a familiar mantra. It was doubled-edged in a stigmatizing condition such as consumption. For the better off in the pre-bacteriology era, a hereditary taint reduced the marriageability of children or siblings. Families would seek to hide tell-tale signs from others and often from the patient in an attempt to encourage them not to lose heart and succumb to the inevitable despondency following such a diagnosis. A good doctor connived, avoiding the diagnosis of consumption or phthisis until there was no other course left open and their patient was beyond hope. Some extended this courtesy to the entry on the death certificate. The new contagiousness could not permit such niceties, particularly among the poorer classes, for they could not be relied upon to behave in such a way as to put the interests of the healthy before their own. Consumption was set to join other reportable diseases as calls were made for its compulsory notification. This was first achieved in New York City, after some considerable 'negotiation'.

In Everyone's Best Interests

Philip's American contemporary Hermann M. Biggs (1859–1923) had also studied abroad. After earning his MD at Bellevue Medical College, New York City, he went to Germany to study, working for some of the time in Koch's laboratory in Berlin (1884–6). Biggs had demonstrated an early commitment to public health, writing his baccalaureate thesis on the government's role in promoting public health and regulating sanitation. He came home inspired by the new bacteriology. Biggs returned to his alma mater at Bellevue, running the Carnegie Laboratory, where bacteriology was quickly applied to public health. He served successively as professor of pathology, materia medica and therapeutics, and the practice of medicine. A busy but committed sanitarian, he was also appointed a consulting pathologist to the city's Department of Health. This administrative work came to dominate the remainder of his career.

In 1889 he co-authored a report (with his colleagues at the department T. Mitchell Prudden and Horace P. Loomis) for the city's Commissioner of Health, Dr Joseph D. Bryant. Biggs and his colleagues optimistically described tuberculosis as 'distinctly preventable' and 'in very many cases distinctly curable' under the programme they advocated: inspection of cattle, mass education, disinfection of the patient's rooms, and compulsory notification of the patient's tuberculous status to the Health Department by attending physicians. Bryant sent out the draft report to a number of physicians and through the newspapers sought to test the opinion of local doctors on its contents. He erred on the side of caution and dropped the final suggestion for notification. An amended version was published as *Rules to be Observed for the Prevention of the Spread of Consumption*. In addition to its reproduction in newspapers such as the *New York Times* on July 10, 1889, ten thousand copies were printed for circulation to medics and interested lay personnel in the city: approximately one copy per 250 people living in the city's five boroughs had they been shared out equally.

Biggs bided his time. In 1893, after successfully implementing measures to prevent the spread of other diseases caused by micro-organisms—cholera, meningitis, and diphtheria—he returned to tuberculosis. A more detailed series of recommendations came out in late 1893. Then in February 1894 he got what he wanted: the thin end of the wedge of compulsory notification. Cattle could already be inspected for tuberculosis all over the state and now the same would apply to all cases of pulmonary tuberculosis diagnosed in the city's public institutions: these must now be reported to the Health Department. Private physicians were urged to comply on a voluntary basis. The department's inspecting manpower was increased and a free sputum examination service instituted at their laboratory. The registry listed its first case on 1 March. Records of living and dead cases were made on printed cards and plotted on street maps in the classic epidemiological style. Elsewhere in the USA others looked on but could not achieve the same ends. Around the world people watched too: *The Lancet* in London called it 'a bold experiment in sanitary regulation'; the German *Zeitschrift für Hygiene* reported both the anti-tuberculosis and anti-diphtheria work and reproduced the sanitary bureaucracy's model paperwork.[17]

While the 1893 legislation had raised relatively little fuss—landlords were cross about the potential costs of disinfection—its subsequent extension to include notification a couple of months later was hotly contested in the press and among the medical fraternity. Biggs referred pugnaciously to the opposers' 'tradition, prejudice and sentiment'.[18] The department sought to tread carefully and to consult with individual practitioners as much as possible to win hearts and minds rather than ruffle feathers. Penalty fines were rarely invoked. Only in the case of low-income patients living in tenements or lodging houses were inspectors sent to patients' homes without the prior consent of their doctor, although this was sought.

In January 1897, empowered by what it perceived as the scheme's success, the Health Department reclassified pulmonary tuberculosis as an 'infectious and communicable disease'. It required every physician to report all cases of this disease which came to their attention within one week of first examining the patient. It had taken seven years from the date of Biggs's initial report. The debate on the absolute role of Koch's bacillus continued in 1890s New York as elsewhere. How much could the disease be attributed to its seed and how much to the soil? With this uncertainty, doctors objected to the breach of confidentiality implicit in compulsory notification and suggested strongly that it wasn't in their patients' best interests. Patients, especially those in the middle and working classes, would deny their symptoms and not seek early diagnosis and treatment if an already stigmatizing disease would make them subject to external scrutiny and control. An extension of the age-old trade-off between the loss of individual liberties for the good of the community was no more appealing at the end of the 19th century. There were practical considerations—most life insurance policies excluded tuberculosis, which left families destitute. Destitute families couldn't pay their doctor's fee.

In the open medical market-place, doctors feared patients were also likely to seek out those who opposed notification or were inclined to offer one of the many more optimistic glosses on their condition: both would lead to a declining practice for a notifying doctor. Fees would be lost if the city or charitable organization took over a patient's care. Family doctors (there were some two thousand practising in this way in the city) felt their livelihoods were under particular threat from the changes ushered in by the new science of bacteriology. There was the growth of public health experts on the one hand and tuberculosis specialists on the other, who were edging them out of the general field of consumption. These financial fears were particularly real during the 1890s as the city's manufacturing sector slumped, unemployment soared, and fees were hard to secure. The major professional doctors' associations, unable to challenge the Health Department at the city level, tried through the State Legislature to scotch Biggs's efforts. They were unsuccessful, although they took up a great deal of his time at the end of the 19th century. Time he would have preferred to spend on developing the institutional aspects of tuberculosis control—hospitals, sanatoria, and dispensaries—to complement the recording and inspection machinery he had put into place.

The kind of slump which hit New York's prosperity during the 1890s had long heightened the fears of working men and women. Tuberculosis would mean time off work without pay. If workers were sick and unable to work, their jobs might be filled by others during periods of abundant labour. During the 19th century, growing numbers of the working classes benefited from participation in self-help organizations such as trade unions and mutual aid and friendly societies. In return for their contributions, members could expect a small sum to tide them over during periods of sickness. Private charitable initiatives might also help but coverage was patchy, tended to be concentrated in large cities, and, as in the case of much mutual aid, did not cover dependants.

In Britain there were moves to recognize that the deserving but sick poor should be spared the necessity of being declared a pauper before they could benefit from medical attention under the Poor Law, sickness being deemed a worthy reason for temporary unemployment. In Germany, which along with America was fast catching up with Britain in its push towards full industrialization, social legislation which protected the worker was introduced as a way of bringing a new statehood to the newly united German-speaking lands and fending off the kind of social unrest that had sparked revolution in 1848 and the Paris Commune in 1871. The German empire's first Chancellor Otto von Bismarck (1815–98) looked at older Prussian precedents, current German industrial relations, and what was happening overseas as he sought to answer calls in the Reichstag for a system of compulsory national insurance.

For many years coalminers' contracts with their employers had included a range of benefits—spa cures, medical treatment, and sickness pay during illness or after an accident, and an invalidity pension if unable to return to work, although these contracts had been overhauled by the final two decades of the 19th century. At the time the 20,000 employees of the metalworking firm Krupp at Essen (one of the largest private companies in Germany) were obliged to contribute to three social funds. First, medical care—to which Krupp also contributed—was paid towards medical expenses and a fairly derisory sickness pay. Another covered accidents, and a third provided for a retirement pension. The workers were not overly fond of these automatic deductions from their wages but this and similar schemes were drawn to Bismarck's attention (he was also a factory owner) by leading industrialists who wished the government to share in the costs of such insurance and maintain a quiescent workforce. In the 1880s three bills were passed to cover sickness (1883), accidents (1884), and old age pensions (1889).

The sickness insurance cover offered a 50 per cent wage for four weeks, rising to two-thirds of the recipient's wage up to a total of thirteen weeks. Typically German wages for factory workers covered by the act (the scheme was subsequently widened) were not much above the cost of living. There was little left over to save against adversity. Even a short period of sickness would tend to put a family into debt. An acute tubercular episode might perhaps be over within thirteen weeks, but workers returning after an enforced break often signed up for overtime, making up for the recent shortfall by overtaxing themselves and increasing the risk of a downward spiral in their heath. The sickness insurance was a safety net of sorts, but in cases of chronic illness it didn't lift the worker much above what he would have been entitled to under the poor law.

Partly to remedy this deficiency, a year later in 1884, Bismarck added a specific clause to the sickness insurance legislation to cover tuberculosis. A worker so diagnosed would now be eligible for a residential stay in the growing number of special institutions being established to treat this disease—tuberculosis sanatoria. A number of factors were probably at work here. It reflected what would become an increasing emphasis on payment in kind as the best use of the money allocated for medical expenses. It also explicitly reinforced the German belief in the sanatorium and the specific medical regime employed there as the best possible treatment for this disease. Just as sickness insurance had its own historical precedents, so too did the use of sanatoria. A special kind of *Kurhaus* (cure house) built either at elevation, in the woods, or by the sea, and advocating either rest or graded exercise in the fresh air, predated Koch's germ theory of tuberculosis. Added to a genuine belief in the curative power of the sanatorium was the recognition that, once removed to it, sick workers did not threaten the health of their colleagues and families. Here, even if a complete cure evaded them, they could be taught to behave as model patients and to manage their condition hygienically for the good of all.

Philip in Edinburgh and Biggs in New York saw the sanatorium as an extension of the dispensary and reporting system each had established. They voiced the hopes of self-conscious progressives in the burgeoning fields of tuberculosis care and prevention. This institutional solution to the tuberculosis problem would be an edifice of the new visibility of tuberculosis as a communicable disease.

VI

⬡

DESIGN FOR LIVING

An Institutional Solution

Glamorized in *The Magic Mountain* at the turn of the 20th century, rendered blackly absurd in *The Rack* towards the end of their reign in the 1950s, sanatoria captured the public imagination. Modernist architects transformed the sanatorium's demands for light and air into buildings that reached beyond their immediate application in curing the sick. The Finn Alvar Aalto (1898–1976) designed not only the functionalist Paimio Sanatorium but its furniture too. The wooden moulded Paimio chairs, now a design icon, were angled so that the breathing of the patients as they rested was as easy as possible. Sanatoria and the sanatorium regime created a little world within a world in the first half of the 20th century. It was a world that would increasingly lose its way and require bolstering by a range of other treatments, but there is no doubt that it began with great confidence.

Sanatoria epitomized attempts to deal with tuberculosis via its own specialized institution. Doctors were soon listing the relative merits of sanatoria in impressive compendia: what sort of soil was the building sited on, how extensive were its grounds, how easily could one reach it by train, how was it furnished, how was the sputum disposed of? So seemingly part of the landscape, they were casually mentioned among the delights of the toboggans and bobsleighs of Davos in the pocket guidebook *Things Seen in Switzerland in Winter* (1926). Here the luxury accommodation, 'with tier upon tier of broad verandas', were 'scattered along the fine promenade which runs through the town, and... on the pine covered mountain slopes above it'. It was not an entirely edifying spectacle: 'this cannot be considered altogether an advantage from the healthy visitors' point of view, as these wonderful hospital-hotels are a somewhat depressing sight.' Yet the balconies, with their prone inhabitants taking the cure, proved that for 'sunshine and pure, dry air Davos has few rivals'. On the up side the continued presence of a tuberculous community brought to the winter sports resort the 'amenities of a civilised centre... with its bands, its promenade—several miles in length—and its English library'.[1] Holiday-makers could come and go, but the floating community of chronic invalids was a constant presence. Some like the writer and sexual freethinker John Addington Symonds (1840–93) remained for many years living the cure rather than merely taking it (he also spent part of each year in Venice). More still stayed in perpetuity, buried in the sizable graveyards, tactfully located away from the main thoroughfares.

Görbersdorf in Upper Silesia, Prussia (now Sokolowsko, Poland) (1859), Nordrach in the German Black Forest (1888), and Davos in the mountains of Grisons in Switzerland (1889) were the sites of the early successful elite sanatoria (there had been a short-lived experiment in 1840 in England). In the countryside, set in large grounds with paths and gardens, the new sanatoria were located in areas renowned for nature and bathing cures. In the mountains others were developed along with the new passion for Alpine winter snow sports. Spa cures continued to be popular with some patients, who found the life of the 'closed' tuberculosis sanatorium not to their taste. Life here was bound by an impressive list of rules to which the patient must adhere, as he or she was taught how to live with the disease, perhaps achieving a cure. Closed sanatoria accepted only tuberculosis cases, were under direct medical supervision, and provided all the necessary therapies on site. If they started small, with a few beds in a simple structure or even a tent, impressive buildings with the characteristic expansive windows, balconies, and verandas generally followed. One sanatorium led to another, as doctors (many of them victims of the disease themselves) set up rival establishments, using their own names and offering personalized versions of the general sanatorium regime. Dr Römpler's Sanatorium (1875) and Dr Weicker's Marienhaus Sanatorium (1888) were close to Dr Brehmer's original Görbersdorf establishment.

Some elite sanatoria opened their doors to admit those of more limited means in suitably segregated areas. Brehmer's admitted 'second-class patients' from 1894 to houses near the main sanatorium and rented rooms in the nearby village. Separate institutions for the struggling professional, poorer members of the middle classes and the working classes also sprang up. Religious groups opened sanatoria for their followers or, as part of a wider remit of charitable care, regardless of faith. The Mount Sinai Sanatorium at Prefontaine near Sainte-Agathe-des-Monts, Quebec, Canada began as a twelve-bedded facility in 1909. It took Jewish tuberculosis patients escaping Montreal's congested city air, increasing in size and widening its intake as funds permitted. Similarly other groups—trades unions, large employers, or cooperative societies—looked to provide facilities.

In 1916 the International Printing Pressman and Assistants' Union added a tuberculosis sanatorium to their technical trade school, retirement home, and headquarters site in the mountains of north-eastern Tennessee, USA. The Metropolitan Life Insurance Company opened a sanatorium for its considerable staff of office workers and field agents in 1913. Care at the purpose-built facility on Mount McGregor, New York State—with its fine views of the famed Revolutionary battlefield of Saratoga—was at the company's expense. A system of underground tunnels allowed discreet removal of the dead to the church and crematorium. In Denmark, the Danish Cooperative Farmers' Association ran the Krabbesholm Sanatorium at Skive by the sea on the Jutland peninsula. Set in wooded grounds, separate buildings for men and women housed patients in multi-bedded rooms. There were two single-bedded rooms in the male house, but it was much more likely that occupants would share a room. As F. R. Walters put it in his encyclopedic *Sanatoria for Consumptives* (1899):

> Sanatoria intended for the poorer classes are usually somewhat different from those where higher charges are expected. Their rooms are less luxuriously furnished; the food is somewhat plainer and less *recherché*; more than one patient are often put into the same bedroom; and a certain amount of the lighter work is expected to be done by those patients who are fit for it.[2]

Sanatorium provision for the working masses followed the differing, often ad hoc arrangements put in place as countries grappled with their tuberculosis problem. Each was a shifting mixture of private benevolence, municipal, parochial, industrial, and state-sponsored efforts. What was mandated at national or local level was often administered by non-governmental organizations. National associations or anti-tuberculosis leagues played an important role in coordinating voluntary efforts against tuberculosis, including raising funds for sanatoria. As the 20th century progressed these national bodies often subsumed smaller pre-existing organizations under their umbrella or established local branches expanding their coverage. France founded her national anti-tuberculosis association in 1891, and the idea snowballed around the globe. Germany followed in 1895, Britain and Belgium in 1898, Portugal, Italy, and Argentina in 1899, Canada in 1900, Denmark and Australia in 1901, the USA and Sweden in 1904, Finland in 1905, Japan in 1908, and Norway and Russia in 1910. Japan might seem the odd one out here. Industrialization and the recent openness at the governmental level to western medicine inspired the country to come to the international table in various ways—not to mention a considerable epidemic of the disease. Tuberculosis control became big charitable business. It would become very visible in the hugely popular sale of Christmas Seals—imitation stamps stuck on to Christmas post. This began in Denmark in 1904, where funds collected were sufficient to open a sanatorium for children in 1911. Other Scandinavian countries and then the USA followed suit.

Germany led the way in the provision of publicly funded institutions after a sanatorium stay was included in the government's social welfare provisions in the 1890s. Three large organizations—the German Central Committee for the Establishment of Sanatoria for Consumptives, the Berlin Brandenburg Association, and the People's Union of the Red Cross—associated with the Imperial Insurance Department took the lead. Various smaller agencies also contributed, such as the government's Forests and Railway departments both of which opened sanatoria for their staff. By 1901 the building mania had borne fruit. At the congress on tuberculosis that year the president of the Imperial Insurance Department reported there were '83 public sanatoria open or ready to open', accommodating '12,000 patients a year'.[3] Britain began a slow expansion of her facilities as the 19th century drew to a close. After the recruitment drive for the Boer War had starkly documented the poor state of health of Britain's military-age men the country looked to improve matters. Part of the solution was the ongoing package of welfare legislation introduced by Lloyd George.

Under the 1911 National Insurance Act the tuberculous were singled out for special provision. This was the only disease for which specialist treatment was available to the insured in the form of 'Sanatorium Benefit' and the only disease in which provision was extended to the insured person's dependants, essentially the wives and children of those working men whose relatively low salaries brought automatic entry into the national scheme. Money was also to be put into research: another exceptional occurrence. Under the financial provisions of the 1911 Finance Act, the Medical Research Committee (subsequently Council) was established to study tuberculosis with an initial annual income of £57,000.

In 1912 Sanatorium Benefit was widened and central government funds were made available to local authorities to cover half the estimated cost of treating non-insured tuberculosis patients in the belief that it was cheaper to attempt a cure rather than to create a permanent invalid on the poor rates. The year 1912 was also when notification was made compulsory in

England, bringing it into line with other infectious diseases. Leasing beds in private institutions met part of the new demand for sanatorium beds. There was a programme of converting existing fever, isolation, and smallpox hospitals owned by local authorities, or large houses sometimes donated by their philanthropic owners. Large windows, sun-rooms, and verandas were added where possible and shelters built in the grounds for the open-air cure. There was a certain timely logic here. The effects of compulsory vaccination had reduced the demands on the smallpox hospitals. Isolation of the infectious tuberculosis patient, when this could not be achieved within the home setting, was a significant part of the rationale for establishing sanatoria.

In the USA the tuberculous doctor Edward Livingston Trudeau (1848–1915) founded the first sanatorium as opposed to an open health resort. During the second half of the 19th century 'health seekers' many of whom were tuberculous 'lungers' crossed America from east to west in search of a healthier place to live. The pioneer settlers had posited the climate of the American west as inherently healthy at mid-century. It became a more accessible if still gruelling journey after the railroad crossed the continent. The tuberculous Robert Louis Stevenson rode the train from New York to California in 1879 in search of his future wife Fanny Osborne, but his delicate health was subject to severe trials en route. He recounted his two-week travails in *Across the Plains* (1892). This would have been a typical experience for many looking for a new, healthier place to live. The most popular destinations were at altitude in the Rocky Mountains in Colorado and in the hot, dry aridity of southern California, Texas, New Mexico, and Arizona, where founding families generally included at least one health seeker.

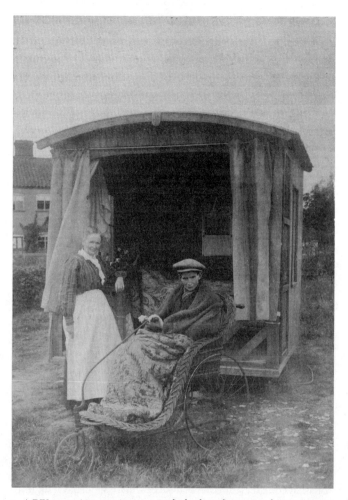

7. A DIY open-air sanatorium cure in the back garden *c.*1900: days were spent in the bath chair, wrapped against the elements and nights sleeping in the chalet. (*Wellcome Library, London*)

Married in 1880, Robert Louis Stevenson and Fanny left the cold damp of San Francisco to honeymoon away from the coastal mists and fogs in the inland mountains of Napa county in California, famous now for its wine. They went for the climate and camped out in a disused hut in the woods. If Stevenson had gone for his health, he conveniently found inspiration for *The Silverado Squatters* (1884). At Saranac Lake in the Adirondack Mountains Trudeau would do much the same without the bother of leaving New York State for the west. He turned his own experiences not into a novel but a sanatorium to which Stevenson would come briefly in the winter of 1887–8. Trudeau had been living a gentle outdoor life at Saranac from the late 1870s after his own tuberculosis responded to this last-ditch attempt to regain his health. Eating a natural diet, hunting from the seat of a rowing boat, and practising a little medicine, Trudeau learned of Peter Dettweiler's version of the sanatorium cure. Dettweiler (1837–1904), a doctor-patient of Brehmer, had opened his own sanatorium in 1876 where he advised an outdoor rest cure, under strict medical supervision. Trudeau realized that he had been running something of a self-experiment but decided to test the principles of Dettweiler's cure more thoroughly using animals.

Trudeau used groups of tuberculosis-inoculated rabbits. The lucky ones he kept in large cages living naturally outdoors on a good diet. He concluded that they did much better than the less fortunate ones confined in a small box in a dark cellar with minimal food. Fresh air and good food worked with tuberculous rabbits. His next experiment was with people. Aware that he might be unable at first to attract paying customers, he decided to offer his facilities cheaply to those of limited means. He teamed up with the New York City doctor Alfred Loomis, a great believer in the potential of the Adirondacks. It was Loomis who had originally suggested Trudeau retreat to the mountains and he would send the tuberculosis patients the experimental facility initially needed.

To his surprise, Trudeau found he was adept at raising funds: $5,000 in the first year. Limiting the Adirondack Cottage Sanitarium to the poor made it an appealing object for philanthropy. Fifteen years after it opened Trudeau's enterprise consisted of several clusters of small cottages, an administration block, a library, a chapel, and an infirmary. Philanthropy helped determine its shape—generous donors liked the idea of having a cottage named in their honour. By 1903 some 1,500 patients had been treated there. Of these 1,066 could be traced and a third reported themselves as 'well'. Two-thirds of those reporting themselves still 'well' had been 'incipient' cases on admission. The cure worked best with those who received an early diagnosis and were admitted immediately.

These selective statistics helped make the Saranac Lake sanatorium a beacon for American tuberculosis control. Almost anyone who was anyone in the tuberculosis field came to talk to Trudeau and to tour the facilities. The rich also came, built their own housing, and placed themselves under the good doctor's care. Ever keen, Trudeau also expanded the facilities to include a research laboratory, further increasing Saranac's prominent position. Initially though, offering a treatment place to the worthy who would otherwise be denied access to a fresh air cure brought in a tractable population. In return for their treatment patients were expected to follow the sanatorium doctors' directions compliantly. Those whose behaviour was 'obnoxious to others' or 'violate[d] the rules of the establishment' would find themselves expelled and back in their nasty tenement cured or not.[4]

Patients were expected to take care of the fixtures, fittings, and themselves. They were to be imbued with a new social responsibility. What they learned about hygiene and moderated living during their cure they were to take home with them and employ as best they could. Adherence to the 'gospel of the germs' was essential, for dirt and morality were closely intertwined. Not following the doctors' orders was a form of moral deviance, which was to be countered by those in authority for the greater good of society. In an era optimistic about the success of sanatorium cures, the power to accept or reject patients was a potent force.

Life Inside

Treatment regimes or cures varied from one establishment to another but the basic principle was as much time spent in the open air as possible. Gone were the closed, heated rooms such as that in which Tom Keats had died. Cold was no longer considered to challenge the lungs. Patients were admitted to the sanatorium, examined by the doctor, and issued with written instructions for conduct during their stay. The first stage of the cure was complete bodily and mental rest to allow the lungs to begin their recovery. Patients were required to take their temperature several times a day, on a daily basis. In the elite sanatoria patients provided their own thermometers, part of the commercial anti-tuberculosis paraphernalia advertised for sale along with spit cups, spittoons, and disinfectants. Temperature charts provided a convenient ready reckoner for determining a patient's progress, how much they might eat or sit up, or how much more strenuous activity was to be permitted. They were supplemented by pulse counts, periodic inspections, weighings, and in some instances X-rays. The highly febrile remained on complete rest, reliant upon the nurse for everything. A mouth-wash replaced the use of the toothbrush. The bedpan had to be used without sitting up or straining—medication would be offered to make sure this happened smoothly. If visitors were discouraged, talking, reading, and hair-brushing were forbidden.

While the rest cure at high altitude or in the dry desert air remained attractive, the new sanatorium movement claimed that effective cures could just as easily be achieved in normal settings with some adjustments. Patients merely needed to be sheltered against excesses of the weather. Those who began the open-air cure in the winter might require 'a short period of acclimatization during which the time and extent of exposure are gradually increased'.[5] After which they would apparently prefer to be outdoors as much as possible: 'A patient who is properly wrapped up with his feet off the ground does not usu-ally feel cold in winter, provided that he is screened from strong wind.'[6] With outdoor lighting installed, staying out after sunset was easy enough. Even the rain was not a problem, for an umbrella and thick rug provided sufficient protection—'so long as the undergarments remain dry and the patient keeps warm, no harm will be done'.[7] Once indoors changing into dry cloth-ing was not essential. The clothes acted as a do-it-yourself 'wet pack', one of the popular hydropathic therapies which over-lapped with the sanatorium era, particularly in Germany. This was just as well since the instructions for patients entering pub-lic sanatoria limited the amount of clothing they might bring in, and frequent changes would have been beyond their resources. Direct exposure to the sun was more of a problem as it tended to increase the risk of fever, hence the covered verandas and large opening windows. Given these rigours the doctors' desire to limit the admission criteria (rarely realized in public sanatoria) to early, afebrile cases began to make very good sense.

Once acclimatized to the outdoor life at rest, the next stage was to gradually increase the amount of activity. This could of course be done without medical supervision, but under the doctor the balance between 'absolute repose or...various degrees of exercise' was struck 'according to definite medical indications'.[8] As the temperature levelled off the amount of permitted activity was gradually increased. Patients could get up to use the toilet; a proper bath replaced the rub-down with a flannel in bed. Meals—considerable in their extent and number, including large quantities of milk to drink—could now be taken in the dining room. 'The discipline of feeding' formed an important part of the cure even in the bed-bound or dyspeptic. Frequently an ordeal for the patient, it was the job of the sanatorium staff to get the food into patients by 'encouragement, moral suasion, even cheerful bullying'.[9] The more febrile the patients, the greater the demands placed upon the staff: another reason why early, afebrile cases were deemed most appropriate for the sanatorium. In the full-price sanatoria Walters recommended one day nurse for every fifteen ambulant patients. For the bed-bound the ratio was lower, one nurse to four patients. In the lower-price sanatoria a single day nurse was expected to cover either a building, or if it was very large at least a floor, which equated to one nurse to thirty or forty patients.

Beyond reclaiming control of one's dignity, the kind of activity patients engaged in when allowed up depended on the sanatorium and their social class. Starting at the top, in Thomas Mann's *Magic Mountain*, life for the sick but otherwise fortunate members of society was a cosseted one in the years before the

First World War. It was a life that for Mann raised questions about the sick role and the moral decay of *fin de siècle* Germany. Describing in delicious detail the precise instructions given to Hans Castorp so he could join his fellow patients in correctly cocooning himself in his blanket for the obligatory rest periods on the balcony was one of the ways Mann highlighted an unhealthy tendency to idleness and indolence. Exercise for the aesthete on the magic mountain involved a timed schedule of walks in the vicinity of the sanatorium with conveniently placed benches.

Alice Clark (1874–1934), part of the wealthy west of England Clark's shoemaking family, also sought to regain her health in high-end sanatoria. Her first short stay was at Nordrach Colonie in the German Black Forest after an operation on her tuberculous neck glands in 1897. She returned home to Somerset in good spirits: 'I am very well and have grown almost too stout, tho' friends are kind enough to say I don't look quite so stout as I weigh! which is 155 lbs.'[10] When her lungs became infected in 1909 she was interred at home on silent bedrest. She made no progress. At the end of the year Alice entered the nearby Nordrach-on-Mendip sanatorium, named for and emulating the regime in the Black Forest, but found it far from acceptable. The medical officer in charge, Dr Rowland Thurnam, was firm with his patients: 'We expect a patient on coming to us to give up his will and inclination for the time being into our hands, and to allow us to have the direction of even the most simple and apparently trivial details of his daily life.'[11] While not expected to work, Alice felt under pressure to do more than she could towards her own personal daily care. Feverish and frail, she rebelled against authority and was eventually allowed to employ her own nurse. Convinced that sanatorium life as lived at the top of the Mendips was making her worse—windows open in sub-zero temperatures and during snowstorms—she begged her mother to let her come home.

Elsewhere in Britain 'graduated labour' had became increasingly popular, especially among those required to deal with the 'industrial class'.[12] For Marcus Paterson, medical officer at the Frimley Sanatorium in Surrey a sanatorium stay need not inculcate habits of laziness and lassitude. Rather than leading to further moral decline (an argument sounded against the use of sanatoria at all), it would make them more resistant to disease. It also prepared patients for an immediate return to their normal working lives on discharge. Paterson was able to underpin his moral and social programme with the immunological theory of autoinoculation, according to which bodily activity released bacterial toxins, and these would stimulate the body's own defences to attack the bacilli. While this could worsen a patient's condition, if carefully controlled by a clinically determined exercise regime, pursued under medical supervision, it would lead to a triumph of the body and arrest of the disease. George Bernard Shaw summed it up neatly in his 1911 play about tuberculosis, *The Doctor's Dilemma*: 'There is at bottom only one genuinely scientific treatment for all diseases, and that is to stimulate the phagocytes.'[13] Patients began by walking. From ten miles a day they moved on to carrying baskets with mould for the extensive lawns, at first a seven-pound basket, followed by a fourteen-pound basket. Next came digging—five minutes on, five minutes off—the initial small spade being replaced with a larger one. In 1910, after five years in charge at Frimley, Paterson reported that 1,674 patients (1,183 men and 491 women) had undergone the graduated labour cure leading to considerable earth and building works. They had prepared and sowed an acre of lawn, constructed a 500,000 gallon reservoir, and laid 650 tonnes of concrete in paths and a subway. The felling of trees—for firewood—threatened to deforest the grounds. As the sanatoria were being established such landscaping was perhaps rewarding but when patients had to resort to digging ditches and then filling them back in any enthusiasm waned. Growing vegetables and keeping poultry harked back to the established model of self-sufficient county lunacy asylums. At the 'Sanatorium for Workers' in Kelling, Norfolk patients carved in wood and made mats for sale.

Not all patients could endure work therapy. Those who deteriorated were placed back on bedrest. A few left in disgust at the regime, arguing they were there to rest, incurring the scorn of the medics. Not all doctors agreed that graduated labour was beneficial. Those with patients of a higher social class worried about how they would find acceptable things for them to do—perhaps games like golf were the answer. After the introduction of a sanatorium cure on the state, funded in part through national insurance deductions, a growing sense of entitlement slowly replaced previous gratitude for charitable care. Patients mostly continued to comply but they complained more. During the First World War rates of tuberculosis temporarily increased in the years of hardship. Soldiers invalided out of the forces for tuberculosis or entitled to an army pension afterwards because of the disease (estimated in 1923 to be some 58,000) were warned they faced a potential loss of benefits should they refuse to do their best to get well.

Reinforcing a patient's desire to get well by doing as they were told continued to be a strong message—one that was supposed to keep them in line inside and to maintain the rules of healthy living on the outside. Betty MacDonald (1908–58) wrote a blackly comic, if poignant, account of her eight months at The Pines sanatorium during 1937–8 in *The Plague and I*. The Pines—a pseudonym for the Firland Sanatorium, just north of Seattle in King county, Washington, USA—aimed to be self-contained. It had a farm, laundry, kitchen and bakery, barber, hairdresser, print shop, and radio service. The self-sufficiency helped to keep costs to a minimum, reducing the burden of the sick on the healthy taxpayers. Finally allowed up for eight hours after following the 'Rules of the Sanatorium' with which she had been issued on arrival, Betty enjoyed typing for the in-house magazine. Such magazines were important for morale and it was more interesting than the endless production of the useless tatted goods made in occupational therapy. The men, when strong enough, were offered classes in the mechanical arts.

More routine work included making the rounds of the bedrest wards with flowers and hot water for washing. Betty was saddened by the deterioration among some of those she had left behind on bedrest. The intense, closed world of the sanatorium was replete with harsh edges. Asked by the Charge Nurse to call and see a woman she had befriended earlier (they had shared their first proper bathing session), Betty reported how the nurse

> tried to prepare me a little telling me that Margaretta was very ill, but nothing she said could have lessened the shock of what I saw. Margaretta's head seemed to have shrunk and become wizened...her hands lay listlessly on the bedcovers like terrible little brown claws. Her voice was completely gone. Only by her large beautiful brown eyes was she recognizable.[14]

Betty also articulated (before Goffman's descriptions of asylum patients) the institutionalizing effects of a sanatorium stay:

It took me the whole summer to learn that you do not dispose of eight and a half months in a sanatorium just by leaving the grounds. I had had to struggle and bleed to adjust to Sanatorium routine and I had to struggle and bleed to adjust back again to normal living. Certain marks of sanatorium life, like the prison pallor, disappeared with time; some, only concentrated effort erased; a few, like the scars from surgery, remained forever.[15]

Beyond Work, Rest, and Play

At eight months, Betty's stay at the Pines was longer than some, shorter than others. As was common in the late 1930s, she also had a surgical operation. Ideally a sanatorium stay should be until apparent cure, but the pressure on sanatorium beds often shortened its duration. Many sanatoria had waiting lists. In Britain in 1913 only 4 per cent (12,000 people) of all cases prescribed the cure could receive such care. As the number of beds expanded so the percentage treated could increase, but in the meantime it was argued that a month in the sanatorium might be enough for educative purposes. In this short time the tuberculous would be exposed to 'discipline and routine'.[16] Such a judgemental jibe reminds that the tuberculous were assumed to be at least partly responsible through their dissolute behaviour for needing a sanatorium place in the first place. They would be taught how to live correctly to improve their condition and carry home with them the schedule of rest and work, instructions for their diet, and the hygienic disposal of their sputum. Cure or more likely arrest—'good health completely restored', 'no T.B. in sputum', would necessarily take longer.[17]

To shorten the stay (on average twelve to fifteen weeks in a public sanatorium in England) and to try to make it more effective, sanatoria began introducing a wider range of treatments to their patients. The long list included many old favourites as well as some new options: dyes; guaiacol and creosote (wood-tar derivatives); plant oils such as the chaulmoograte from India; morrhuates—the fatty acids of that old staple cod liver oil; arsenicals and metals such as copper, gold, mercury, cadmium, and manganese. Elite sanatoria had always offered extras at a price. In the interwar years public sanatoria widened their therapeutic assistance. This brought career opportunities for sanatorium doctors and surgeons. It also blurred the boundaries between sanatoria and other institutions involved in the battle against the disease.

Provision of additional therapies was a tilt towards the open critics of the sanatorium movement. In England, the Australian William Camac Wilkinson rounded on the optimism surrounding the new tuberculosis provisions in 1911. He cited disturbing follow-up studies from thirty-one sanatoria in Germany: four years after discharge 80 per cent were either dead or invalids. Halliday Sutherland, formerly medical superintendent at the Westmorland Sanatorium in coastal Cumbria, gave much the same sort of figures for patients treated in England during 1914; by 1920 80 per cent of them were dead. Rather than sanatoria Wilkinson promoted tuberculin. He had been in England since 1909 and had treated Alice Clark after she fled the regime at Nordrach-on-Mendip.

Tuberculin had been Robert Koch's attempt at a specific treatment. His reputation as discoverer of the *Tubercle bacillus* lent obvious support to his announcement in August 1890 in Berlin of a new treatment. The tuberculous importuned Koch, seeking access to the clinicians administering his tuberculin, or badgered their own doctors to obtain the magical fluid. It was released more widely in November. Early high-profile patients included the ailing niece of Britain's first surgical lord, Joseph Lister. He took her with him when he travelled to Berlin to observe at first hand Koch's breakthrough. Lister had pioneered the application of germ theory in surgery, reducing the mortality from post-surgical infection. Such faith from one bacteriologist to another was compelling. Koch's initial results appeared to be a series of sensational recoveries. Although it did not dim his support, Lister's niece was not among the lucky ones. She apparently suffered an accelerated decline. The tuberculin, far from curing her, brought on a catastrophic fever and illness— what would later be understood as a strong allergic reaction.

The early 'cures' could not be replicated beyond those closely associated with Koch. This small, apparently successful, group included Koch's son-in-law Eduard Pfuhl, which fuelled the antagonism. Koch's subsequent disclosure about what tuberculin actually was brought more disdain. Tuberculin was not an antibacterial drug, but a potion made from the cultures of the bacillus, dissolved in glycerine. After his discovery of the germ Koch had begun looking for a safe internal disinfectant—a chemical that would kill bacteria in the body without damaging healthy tissues. After his search failed—some success in the test-tube, but not in the body of experimentally infected guinea pigs—he turned towards an immunological solution.

Vaccine therapy had been very successful in the hands of Koch's great French rival Louis Pasteur, whose rabies vaccine had grabbed the world's attention in 1885. On the basis of his animal experiments, Koch believed tuberculin did not attack the bacilli but the tubercle tissue where the bacteria were lodged, so that the safe pathological stage of caseation and necrosis was reached quickly. In tissue rendered into a dry cheese-like state the bacteria could not feed or multiply and eventually died: 'a bacteriological variation of a scorched earth strategy'.[18] This was particularly visible in tuberculosis of the skin—lupus vulgaris—where nodules and ulcers are readily evident. The tuberculous tissue would become inflamed, slough off, and be replaced by healthy scar tissue. Inside the body, the same was presumed to happen. Koch reported that in early cases of pulmonary tuberculosis 'cough and expectoration generally increased a little at the first injection, then grew less and less, and in the most favourable cases entirely disappeared … within four to six weeks patients under treatment for the first stage of phthisis were all free from every symptom of disease'.[19] Treatment involved a course of tuberculin injections of increasing strength, say 2 to 8 mg rising to 4,000 mg over a three-week period. Each was to be given after the systemic reaction—high fever, chills, aching, possibly vomiting—and local tissue reactions had subsided.

While he was enthusiastic about its effect on bone, skin, and early pulmonary cases, Koch was chary about the likely success in advanced pulmonary cases. He also warned that he was unsure about his product's active life—how long it remained fully potent—and this was certainly a problem. Others were more sweepingly critical. Rudolf Virchow challenged Koch's idea that the necrotic stage was the end of the infection. Instead he called attention to the fresh new tubercles arising at the edges of the necrotic tissue—the infection was ongoing. A worrying tendency to relapse after initial success backed this up. In some cases after treatment patients sickened dramatically and died soon after. Clinician Ottomar Rosenbach called the induced febrile episodes highly dangerous side effects. Was the body's severe reaction indeed a positive one as Koch claimed? It seemed in fact 'that large doses cause damage…whereas small doses don't help'.[20] As the number of failures grew, and suspicion that Koch had kept the precise nature of his tuberculin secret for financial gain, mass interest subsided.

The principle of tuberculin, however, retained a small if dedicated following. Koch returned to the fray more than once, developing in 1901 the so-called 'new tuberculin'. Once tuberculin's basic nature was understood there was considerable scope for developing alternative preparations, attenuating bacteria from different sources and experimenting with dosage and injection schedules. Friedrich Franz Friedmann (1876–1953) used cultures of bacilli originally taken from the lungs of turtles housed at the Berlin zoo in 1902. He began reporting favourable results from 1904. International interest in the 'turtle cure' accelerated late in 1912 when Friedmann rushed a sample of his vaccine to the Public Health Department in Berlin. He asked for public trials, but was essentially seeking an official endorsement of his unpatented remedy to thwart his former assistant, a Dr Piorkowski, who had betrayed him by giving some of the vaccine away. Dr A. B. Reid of Pittsburgh, USA came to Germany on a desperate mission to try to save his wife, bringing with him an unnamed companion who wanted the potentially lucrative 'honor of introducing Dr. Friedmann's remedy in the United States'.[21] Friedmann was extremely keen to protect his cure. He had already received an offer of $1,000,000 if he cured ninety-five out of a hundred patients in America. Businessman Charles E. Finlay had only one stipulation: that the hundred would include his son-in-law Rex Lees Paris currently at the Saranac Lake sanatorium.

Friedmann crossed the Atlantic in February 1913 and began treating patients from his hotel. He struck up a relationship with Moritz (or Morris) Eisner, head of the Standard Distributing Company, which sold such things as Carlsbad Mineral Waters. Concerns were aired in the *New York Times* about Friedmann's legal right to charge for his remedy and its efficacy as inoculated patients failed to recover, worsened, and in some cases died soon after treatment. Meanwhile he was negotiating in lawyers' offices and hotel rooms. Sensational headlines in late April revealed Friedmann had rejected plans for free treatment for the poor. Instead he planned a network of fee-paying Friedmann institutes. The syndicate headed by Eisner would pay Friedmann $125,000 in cash and $1,800,000 in stock in the thirty-six eponymous institutes as they were established. The next day Friedmann reaffirmed his commitment to free treatment for those who could not pay but the distribution rights to his cure had been decided. Then Maurice A. Sturm, a hotel doctor, who had assisted Friedmann by treating some of the early patients, claimed to have the secret of the cure and threatened to break the monopoly. Friedmann was accused by the authorities of not properly completing the treatment of some patients and not complying with government requests to treat patients under their scrutiny. Crowds gathered at the entrance to a hospital with their tuberculous children in carriages. A mother threw herself in the path of his car desperate for treatment for her 9-year-old son.[22] In late May the Board of Health in New York called a halt to the 'turtle cure' in the city, writing a new clause for the Sanitary Code, which outlawed 'the use of living bacterial organisms in the inoculation of human beings for the prevention of or treatment of disease'.[23] Eisner, lamely hubristic to the end, encouraged New Yorkers to attend the Friedmann Institute in Providence, Rhode Island, beyond the state boundary. The turtle cure, with its advocates and disparagers, took its place

beside other vaccine therapies. Friedmann sailed for Europe in
June with at least $30,000.

While such large sums of money had swirled around the turtle cure others championed tuberculin for exactly the opposite
reason: manufactured locally, it was cheap and could be administered through the existing dispensary system. Robert Philip in
Edinburgh supported this in Scotland. Sanatorium beds were
scarce, and patients' lives were severely disrupted during their
institutionalization. Many more could be treated at the dispensary. Ideally it was possible to treat early cases with a series of
tuberculin injections while they continued their normal working lives. In reality the dispensary had to be open—as did happen in the interwar years—outside of working hours. The
possibility of a series of tuberculin injections would encourage
those with incipient disease to come forward, preventing their
health deteriorating and countering further spread of the disease. Camac Wilkinson's Tuberculin Dispensary League in
London pushed for this well into the 1920s, but while he had
some financial support, local general practitioners resented the
intrusion. The usual dispensary fare—education, inspection,
disinfection, bacteriological analysis, and distribution of milk,
cod liver oil, and sputum flasks—were less of a threat to the
doctors' income.

Tuberculin and similar vaccines also made an appearance at
the outpatients' departments of the specialist voluntary
hospitals—charitable institutions for the deserving poor. Four
consumption and chest hospitals had been founded in London
in the 19th century as the voluntary hospital movement
expanded, with specialist institutions devoted to a particular illness or part of the body. Consumptives, as chronically sick,
were unlikely to gain admission to general voluntary hospitals

where they either stayed too long or died—outcomes which involved too much nursing, blocked beds, and ruined the discharged 'cured' or 'improved' rates. Even at the first and most famous of the specialist hospitals, the Brompton (founded in 1841) the emphasis was on short-stay acute patients. After 1904 the longer-stay patients went to its country outpost—the Frimley sanatorium where graduated labour was promoted. The outpatients' department offered much the same kind of function as a dispensary and conducted a brisk business. Brompton saw upwards of 200 patients a day, who shuffled along the benches in the waiting room 'coughing, hawking, intermittently disappearing down a corridor upon a sharp summons to a test or examination'.[24]

Surgical Solutions

In the interwar period outpatients' departments and dispensaries also began offering 'gas' refills on a regular basis. This unlikely-sounding procedure was the maintenance stage in one of the leading surgical operations for pulmonary tuberculosis—artificial pneumothorax—one of several kinds of lung collapse therapy. These invasive procedures aimed to rest the lung while allowing the body housing it to be off the rest and graduated exercise cures more quickly. Bacteriological evidence from sputum tests indicated that the collapsed lung was less likely to shed bacilli, endowing this therapy with an importance beyond each individual case.

Chance observations—that sometimes patients with a lung injury would heal at greater speed when a spontaneous collapse of the lung took place—ought to apply to a lung compromised by tubercular lesions, suggested James Carson in Liverpool in the 1820s. Some sixty years later the Italian Carlo Forlanini (1847–1918) developed a reliable method of admitting air into the pleural cavity. This sac envelops the lung. Inside this closed space the lung is held tight against the chest wall by the negative pressure in the cavity. The introduction of air or an inert gas into the cavity allows the pressure inside and out to equalize and the lung collapses inwards onto itself. So long as the level of the introduced air is maintained in the pleural cavity—hence the 'refills'—the lung will remain quiescent. The medical director told Betty MacDonald before her pneumothorax that 'collapsing a lung was like putting a splint on a broken leg'.[25] The refills weekly, monthly, and then six-monthly could last up to five years or until the lung was healed. Once the lesions were declared sufficiently healed the refills ceased and the lung became operative again. In reality the collapsed lung often healed with scarring, becoming a 'chronic fibroid' case. Such a lung would never regain its original capacity, but it might stop exuding bacteria into the sputum.

The familiar refrain of greater success in early cases applied to pneumothorax. In more advanced cases there was a greater tendency for the lung to be attached to the surrounding tissues. Such adhesions would impede collapse and preparatory cauterization to cut through them would be required. Early cases were usually restricted to one lung only, which was obviously better than when both (a bilaterial case) lungs were involved, but it was still possible to rest the most affected lung. If this was successful—the sputum dried up and lost its bacilli, and weight loss and fever were not too severe—then the first lung could be re-expanded and the other one collapsed. Collapse was achieved by simply inserting a needle into the pleural cavity. Greater control of the amount of introduced air was achieved by a water manometer (an air pressure monitor), first used by Christian Saugman at the Vejleford sanatorium, Denmark. At the beginning of Betty's first collapse the nurse

> told me to lie on my back with my left arm above my head, then painted the entire upper left half of me with mercurochrome.
>
> The Medical Director was washing his hands over in the corner... when he had finished the nurse handed him a pair of rubber gloves, which he put on without speaking. Then he poked me experimentally in the ribs, looked at my X-rays, examined my case history and said, 'Yell if you want to but don't flinch!'
>
> I felt the prick of the hypodermic needle, just under my left breast, then an odd sensation as though he were trying to push me off the table, then a crunchy feeling and a stab of pain. 'There now', the Medical Director said, as he attached the end of what looked like a steel knitting needle to a small rubber hose connected to two gallon-fruit jars partially filled with a clear amber fluid. The nurse put one jar higher than the other and I waited frantically for my breathing to stop and suffocation to start. There was no sensation of any kind for a few minutes then I had a pulling, tight, feeling up around my neck and shoulder. The doctor, said, 'I guess that's enough for to-day', took the needle out, slapped a bandage on me and I got down from the table, dizzy with relief.[26]

In the evening Betty experienced a few after effects: 'sharp, knifelike pains in my chest and I had spit up a little blood'.[27] She was advised that the chest pain, which continued for another seventy-two hours, was caused by the adhesions gradually tearing loose; the blood was 'probably' from her nose. The nurse opined that 'I was most fortunate to be able to take pneumothorax', which had been delayed until a shadow on her right lung

had cleared up with the rest cure. She had been in the sanatorium for a month and two days. Betty did not suffer any more
serious complications. Air embolism—a bubble of air introduced into a vein—was potentially fatal. As late as 1959 dispensary staff were advised to have a back door for the discreet
removal of unconscious patients: 'In all places where pneumothorax treatment is done tragedies occur.'[28] Pleural shock could
also render patients unconscious, as the needle appeared to
stimulate 'nerves in the pleura giving rise to temporary failure
of the heart'.[29] In subcutaneous emphysema air was accidentally
introduced under the skin. Patients felt a 'crackling sensation'
and experienced swelling, which could spread alarmingly
upwards to the face. They were advised to press a hand over the
needle puncture whenever they wanted to cough to stymie this
backflow of air. Betty was also lucky because the doctor was
working with her chest X-ray in front of him and the extent of
her collapse was subsequently assessed by use of the fluoro-
scope. This X-ray technique allowed the doctor to watch her
breathing rather than taking a still image. Even in the late 1930s
doctors in Britain were often still working 'blind'.

If this all sounds rather rough and ready, it was. Pneumothorax was usually performed by medically rather than surgically
trained sanatorium staff. It was a way for this somewhat lowly
group of medical professionals to increase their status. It was a
chance to show that they were really doing something for their
patients. Other kinds of collapse required the skills of a surgeon
and the use of anaesthesia beyond a local novocaine injection.
In cases prevented from the standard collapse because of the
extensive pleural adhesions the pleura could be stripped from
the chest wall. This formed a pocket, which could be filled with
air or sterile oil. A thoracoplasty involved removing a portion

of the ribs to allow a permanent lung collapse. Without the support of the ribs the body caved in on itself, leaving the patient with a rested lung and a disfigured body. The goal was to remove seven or eight ribs, but it was often done two or three at a time in a series of operations. Should they be fortunate to survive, many developed long-term respiratory problems because of their reduced lung capacity. A follow-up of some of the estimated one million Japanese patients who had undergone chest surgery from 1950 to 1960 provided distressing evidence of this mass mutilation done for what at the time were considered to be good reasons.[30]

Crushing the phrenic nerve—phrenicotomy—was performed though a small incision just above the collarbone. The phrenic nerves emerge from the vertebral column in the neck. Interrupting their communication with the muscular diaphragm causes this tissue to rise up, in some cases by as much as 14 cm, compressing and thus resting the lower part of the lung. Some doctors used this operation as the primary means of collapse, where there were lesions low in the lung. In others it was employed after pleural adhesions prevented pneumothorax. Nerve crush was often used with pneumoperitoneum—inserting air into the abdominal peritoneal cavity to force up the diaphragm—where the more major operation to remove the ribs was inadvisable. The crush was intended to be a short-term—a three- to six-month—disablement of the diaphragm. Not infrequently—'figures vary from 6 to 10 per cent'—the diaphragm was permanently disabled.[31] Should this actually be the desired result the more radical phrenicectomy involved removal of a segment of the phrenic nerve.

A review undertaken in 1947 in the USA attempted to evaluate the effects of nerve crush when it enjoyed a resurgence in the immediate postwar years. The authors looked as systematically as they could at a series of X-rays and concluded that the effects on shrinking or closing cavities in the lungs were limited. In their opinion the drying up of active lesions was better than with pneumothorax. They gave cautious support to the combined effects of nerve crush and pneumoperitoneum. Early cases gave better results, but, as they acknowledged, they also tended to heal spontaneously. The authors had to admit that their comparisons had been hampered by difficulties in comparing like with like. There were considerable differences in the timing of operations and the patient's condition before treatment. Case reports, as opposed to properly conducted trials with statistical evaluations, dominated the tuberculosis literature. There was still an overriding emphasis on doing something perhaps for the doctor as well as the patient:

> In patients with extensive bilateral disease, in whom bedrest produced little or no change, and where collapse therapy was impossible, pneumoperitoneum succeeded in improving their morale in a large measure. There was gain in weight, lessening of cough and expectoration, and occasionally slight changes noted on x-ray in the nature of improvement...such a mode of therapy has a very useful function in psychologic problems related to the tuberculous, particularly when the patient observes that despite deterioration of his condition or lack of progress no treatment other than bedrest is given him.[32]

The growth in surgery was part of a transition from the 'sanatorium era' towards the 'hospital era' of tuberculosis treatment.[33] Surgery increased the sense that sanatoria were developing into modern specialist hospitals, with a range of skilled staff who were empowered by what they could do for the patient, rather than what they could teach the patient to do for themselves. Sanatorium nurses were often hard to recruit; some were ex-patients who were used to the routines. It was hoped that career nurses who gained experience with thoracic surgery would enjoy a higher profile and help raise this branch of the profession. Many sanatoria were necessarily constrained to adapt space or to add surgical units to existing buildings. Where new buildings were possible, they looked, as many new hospitals, more like a contemporary office block, apart from the oversized windows.

The Royal Edward Institute in Montreal, Canada moved to a new site in 1933 when the old building, a converted three-storey house, was demolished to make way for a railway station. The Royal Edward had begun as a dispensary, then moved into providing a limited number of day spaces for the rest cure. Planned by an architect with experience in both hospital and school design, the new building housed a range of tuberculosis services. As well as offering the traditional sunlight and fresh air via the large opening windows, there were also a surgical suite and dedicated space for diagnostic X-ray equipment. Space was set aside for 'broader social technologies'. Visiting nurses were based here, returning each evening after completing their schedule of contract-tracing and supervision of those practising the rest cure at home. There were always far more of these doing the best they could in limited circumstances: sleeping in beds placed next to or even partially through open windows or in jerry-built shelters on roof tops.

In its new premises the Royal Edward became an affiliated institution of McGill University. In 1941 the McGill hospitals streamlined surgical care of tuberculosis by sending all cases to the Royal Edward. A new operating room was added in the internal reorganization (the school had closed). In this fully equipped space, more dramatic thoracic surgery would take place. Internal operations within the chest, the removal of a part of the diseased lung (lobectomy) or the whole lung (pneumonectomy), joined the repertoire. In the new hospital era many patients were both dosed with the new antibiotics and underwent surgery as part of a combined cure, until the use of surgery faded in the wake of the unalloyed success of the drugs. Experience with tubercular patients would then help to train a new generation of specialist chest surgeons. In the second half of the 20th century, as the number of tuberculosis patients continued to decline and facilities were freed up, they were able to transfer their skills to other serious conditions within the thoracic cavity such as lung cancer, but that lay in the future.

For the moment we leave this transition delicately poised on the cusp and take a step back to follow a different route to those declining numbers. Many of the sanatoria that have featured here were exclusively adult places. It was perhaps hard enough for the staff to maintain discipline between the sexes without taking care of children. Yet it was in the sanatorium era that the plight of the young tuberculous came to the fore as eugenic fears for the health of the nation and the threat of tuberculosis as a racial poison both reared their ugly heads.

VII

TUBERCULOSIS AND THE HEALTH OF THE RACE

'Looking for the Angels'

At the start of the 20th century children posed a special tuberculosis problem. With the ascendancy of germ theory the tubercle bacillus was understood to be the cause of their chronically diseased joints and intestines, and the dramatic infections in the tissues lining the skull. Debilitated children often faced a lifetime of ill health as poorly adults. The feeble in body were a drain on the emerging communal systems of health care and social insurance. They could also pass on their enfeeblement to the next generation—the great fear of the social Darwinists—and produce their own weakling children in an ever-downward spiral.

Countries began to register growing concerns about the health of their population. Military and industrial strength were at stake. Fear of degeneration and desire for racial hygiene affected attitudes to the tuberculous child and what it might become. In a similar way non-whites were often seen as 'children'. The other races, especially the subjects of European tropical empires and African and Native Americans in the USA also challenged ideas of racial health. What was the relationship between ethnicity and tuberculosis and how should it be managed? Should those suffering from this 'disease of civilization' be helped to acclimatize or left to die out, so that only the strongest survived? If germ theory had begun to explain the role of the 'seed', the reaction of the 'soil'—the immunological response of the host to this invasion—had to be gauged afresh. These were subjects where opinion was strong, substantive evidence weak, and attitudes often unpleasant.

As with the adults the special institution led the way in defining care of the tuberculous child in the early 20th century. A few adult sanatoria had included facilities for various aspects of childhood tuberculosis. The original Royal Edward dispensary in Montreal, Canada opened an open-air school in 1912, where children were taught all year round on the veranda. Some sanatoria included beds for children. The Firland in Seattle had a special building, the Josef House, which took in those up to the age of 15. Some had tuberculosis; others were being treated prophylactically because they came from homes with a tuberculous relative. The Josef also cared for children whose mothers had been admitted to the main sanatorium so they could undergo their cure. Betty MacDonald's children were fortunate and stayed at home, cared for by her female relatives. The Craig-y-nos sanatorium in Wales, housed in a converted mock castle, opened in 1922. There were in-patient beds for adult pulmonary cases and for children who mostly suffered non-pulmonary tuberculosis. Elsewhere dedicated facilities evolved in parallel to cater for tuberculous children, including those at risk, but not yet sick, the so-called pre-tubercular.

Children's requirements were different because they tended to suffer much more from extrapulmonary tuberculosis. This is related partly to diet—the greater consumption of raw milk—leading to infection with the bovine form of the tubercle bacillus. Acute abdominal tuberculosis killed quickly, but a slow spread from a primary focus in the alimentary tract into the mesenteric and abdominal glands was a more protracted process. Such children would be small, wasted, and suffer from periodic fever. If the tissues lining the abdomen were compromised—tuberculous peritonitis—fluid could flow into the peritoneal cavity, causing significant swelling. The grossly distended abdomen in concert with the otherwise emaciated body made a wretched picture.

Tuberculous meningitis was a fast killer and could appear without much other evidence of infection. As the disease affected the tissues surrounding the spinal cord including the cranial nerves the little victim's eyes became fixed and dilated as if staring upwards, 'looking for the angels' to take them to their rest.[1] Or so a doctor might tell the desperate parents unable to relieve their distress in any other way. The acuteness of disease tailed off in children aged between 3 and 15, and the tendency to adult-like pulmonary disease increased as they grew older.

Children could also become infected through their lungs. The importance of this route was unravelled in the 1920s and 1930s. A study for the Medical Research Council showed that when the primary infection was in the abdomen (one-third of the cases), bovine bacilli were found in 82 per cent of the cases. When the primary infection was in the lungs (two-thirds of cases), 97 per cent of the bacilli found were of human origin.[2] Infants under 3 years were extremely vulnerable to infection and died quickly either of an acute disease of the lungs or a generalized (miliary) tuberculosis after the bacilli spread through the bloodstream.

If they were infected in the same way as adults—via their lungs from inhaled bacilli—children succumbed to an acute infection or coped with minimal outward evidence of illness. In this case their lungs contained a highly characteristic lesion— a Ghon focus—named after the pathologist Anton Ghon (1866–1936). Better understanding of this lesion and assessment of its frequency led to the realization that the airborne route was significant in childhood disease. Should the disease not be contained and bacilli spread within the body, the glands and bones were commonly affected. Swollen neck glands were visible, as was the ulceration of the skin. These benefited from the work of the Danes Niels Finsen (1860–1904) and Sophus Bang (1866–1950), who pioneered the therapeutic use of artificial ultraviolet light. Finsen founded his medical light institute in 1896 in Copenhagen. He won the Nobel Prize in 1903. Finsen lamps became popular where funds permitted their use. Children wearing protective goggles and not much else would be illuminated in special rooms. Cheaper quartz mercury lamps were good for small areas of the skin. Tuberculosis in the bones and joints was hidden at first, but as the chronic destruction proceeded, children became bent and distorted, and cried out such was the pain of the accompanying muscle spasms.

The revolutionary developments of the second half of the 19th century—anaesthesia, antisepsis, then asepsis—allowed surgeons time in the operating theatre to practise more conservative surgery. In the case of tubercular joints this involved scraping out and draining joints, which previously might have been left untreated or simply amputated. It was a slow process and required considerable after-care. The surgeon Robert Jones (1857–1933) opened one of the first orthopaedic hospitals for children at Heswall near Liverpool in 1898. Many of his young patients were suffering from tuberculosis. Such institutional facilities for the treatment of 'crippled children' expanded. Some began to offer basic education and perhaps training in a trade to their long-stay patients. There was an expansion too in the equipment used to treat these kids—the Bradford frame, Whitman frame, Gauvain's spinal board, Gauvain's back-door splint, Pyrford frame, Thomas splint for the knee and hip. Named for their inventors, they were designed to straighten and support limbs and backs as they healed. Extension techniques—a slow pulling to relax the contracted muscles—used weights and pulleys or the counterweight of the body. Traction aimed to keep the child's joints movable. Such care could obviate the need for surgery altogether, although abscesses needed aspiration.

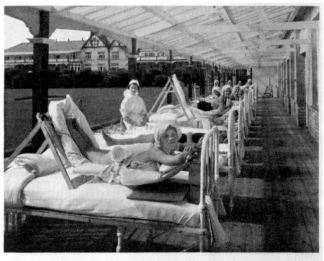

SENIOR GIRLS—SURGICAL CASES.
Correction of deformity being carried out by hyper-extension in plaster.
Children are accommodated with due regard to age as well as to physical condition.

8. Sunshine, fresh air and surgery for the 'senior girls' at the Stannington Sanatorium, Morpeth, Northumberland. The first British children's tuberculosis sanatorium (1907), funded by a local charity, it used immobilizing plaster casts and frames to treat bone tuberculosis. (*Wellcome Library, London*)

In addition to the metal frames, plaster of Paris casts were also used to immobilize affected body parts. In both cases rest of the diseased bony area, until signs of active disease had ceased, underpinned the treatment rationale, just as it did in pulmonary cases. Shells, jackets, and splints could cover extensive areas. A jacket used for Pott's disease in the cervical region—involving the bones of the neck—would continue up and over the head, leaving only the face and ears exposed. In the body-encasing jackets windows were cut to allow the chest and abdomen to expand as the patient breathed and after eating. As for the other necessaries of life, a protective sheet of rubberized fabric or oiled silk was used on the edges of the cast to protect against contamination with urine or faeces. Children were admonished to be 'cleanly in their habits' and nurses instructed to check their charges against 'a peculiar smell'—the sign of a plaster sore.[3]

Nurses took pride in the care they offered: 'between supper time and before we went off duty, we'd do skin care to prevent pressure sores.' The reasons quickly became obvious: 'children with TB hip were in plaster round their waist and down their leg. Sometimes the plaster would dig into their skin—into their bottom usually. I remember one little boy was crying one day and wouldn't tell me what was wrong. When we eventually turned him over, the plaster was cutting into his bottom.'[4] Peter Wagstaffe spent five years lying prone at the Craig-y-nos sanatorium:

> I was in a splint with my legs apart and straps across my chest. You could only move your head and arms ... We used to make up our own games. We were in a row in beds and we used to play cricket. We'd have a book on one locker—that was the wicket, and we'd have a patient about three beds

away with a big ball of newspaper rolled up on a string. He'd bowl the ball to us and try to hit the wicket, and if we could hit it the length of four beds, it was four runs, and six beds it was six runs.

When he was finally allowed out of bed, Peter was fitted with a calliper but had to return to the sanatorium to have his hip locked after six months at home. Treatment in a plaster cast could be continued with a celluloid jacket, which was worn to try and prevent further deformity once the child was up.

...Better than Cure

'Prevent' is surely the operative word. Since the turn of the twentieth century activists who wished to save children from a fate similar to Peter's wanted to tackle tuberculosis before it struck. Worries about tuberculous children were a specific part of the more general concerns about national degeneration at the end of the 19th and into the early 20th century. In France the loss of the Franco-Prussian war fuelled fears about the nation's future. Attempts to redress the falling birth rate and to take care of those children already born spurred various initiatives. In 1888 the L'Oeuvre des Enfants Tuberculeux was established to offer free treatment for any tuberculous child in Paris. After assessing the children L'Oeuvre des Enfants used existing facilities outside of Paris at Ormesson, Villiers-sur-Marne, and Berck-sur-Mer to provide a combination of fresh country and seaside air and the usual treatments. The hospital at Villiers, nine miles from the centre of Paris, had the children out during the day while at night they slept in rooms artificially ventilated with the popular inhalants creosote, turpentine, or eucalyptus.

In 1902 Jacques-Joseph Grancher (1843–1907) founded L'Oeuvre de Preservation de l'Enfance Contre la Tuberculosis. Grancher had been a long-time advocate of the infectious nature of tuberculosis and this inspired the thrust of L'Oeuvre Grancher, as it subsequently became known. Grancher claimed that the morbidity of children who remained in tuberculous households ran at 60 per cent and mortality at 40 per cent. This was enough to inspire the charity to step in before children needed hospitalization. One of its more dramatic measures was to identify and farm out at-risk children aged between 3 and 10 from their diseased urban homes to the salubrious countryside, where they would live with farming families. Many remained with their foster families after they passed the official returning age of 13. The system was extended back to pregnant tuberculous women who apparently agreed to give up their children after they were born. If the father was tuberculous and would not enter a sanatorium the mother was also encouraged to part with her child. One can only guess at the moral or other forms of persuasion used, and the pain. A report in 1923 referred to the records of 2,300 Grancher children, among whom there had been only seven cases of tuberculosis and two deaths from tubercular meningitis, statistics which naturally satisfied the movement's leaders.[5]

Germany might have beaten the French in 1871 but the newly unified country was keen to continue to build up its military strength by taking care of tomorrow's soldiers from an early age. The instruments of state welfare crept over the threshold to dictate aspects of family life. Alarmist estimates suggested that between 3 and 5 per cent of all schoolchildren in German cities missed their classes because of sickness, stoking fears over the level of incipient tuberculosis. School nurses began conducting routine assessments of the pupils' ill health, while sports programmes were initiated to promote better health.

By 1900, as in Scandinavia, Germany was using its North and Baltic Sea coasts for seaside sanatoria for at-risk children. Only small numbers could attend Germany's four residential institutions and they closed down in the winter. In 1904 a charitable initiative in the Berlin suburb of Charlottenberg sought to bring the benefits of the open-air life closer to the city for twelve months of the year. When a local business loaned a five-acre site for an outdoor school, a women's group—the Vaterländische Frauenverein—found the money to bring the children from the inner city, and provide special furniture such as reclining chairs. The government paid for the teachers. The children slept at home but spent eleven hours a day, seven days a week, at the school. While the weather was fine the children learned and played outside. Lightly dressed to make the most of the sun's health-giving rays, the children ate five meals a day and had lessons for only three hours to avoid overtaxing their strength. Their progress was measured by weight gain; those who failed to gain the extra pounds were sent to the doctor for a medical inspection. The results were sufficiently pleasing for the government to copy the model across Germany. Overseas visitors carried it home with them.

In the United States they coined a new word—the preventorium—to describe their fresh-air facilities for the pre-tubercular. The first, a tented colony in the beach resort of Coney Island near New York City (1904), attracted attention from wealthy holiday-makers. Permanent buildings replaced the tents at Sea Breeze and the idea spread on the east and west coasts and around the large urban areas of the Midwest. Initially taking youngsters of about 5 and upwards, some opened crib wards for nursing infants. Preventoria were replete with the values of the Progressive Era, summed up in a song from the institution at Farmingdale, New Jersey:

P is for prevention much better than cure
R is for rest in the open pure air
E is for evils of dirt, and foul air,
V is for vices that lead to despair
E education, improving the mind
N stands for nurses, so helpful and kind
T is for toothbrush, used three times a day
O is for outings, fresh air and play
R means refuse to touch soiled cloth or towel
I means infection from drinking-cup foul
U is for us—most sincerely we pray
M is for much strength to do service each day
P–R–E–V–E–N–T–O–R–I–U–M (repeated several times getting
    louder each time)[6]

Inspirational as these measures might have seemed to their providers, and lonely and isolating for the many children and parents separated on advice or orders, they could reach only a limited number. In the 1920s, after an aggressive building pro-gramme, the American National Association for the Prevention of Tuberculosis estimated there were still only 2,783 preven-torium beds nationwide. Year-round facilities were augmented with places in dedicated summer camps for the pre-tubercular, offering sports facilities and nourishing food in the sunshine. In the public schools educational programmes began in the 1910s. Later the National Tuberculosis Association also sponsored the creation of the cartoon characters Huber the Tuber and Tommy Tubercle, whose antics aimed to educate while they entertained. All chimed with the general enthusiasm for using a range of institutional solutions to solve social and medical problems. More expansive preventive measures came from a different tack.

Calf with a Cough

The movement to provide a clean milk supply predated the concerns with preventing tuberculosis, but was energized by the disturbing levels of the *tubercle bacillus* in what should have been a pure natural product. Knowledge that the presence of these organisms in milk could infect vulnerable children added urgency to cleansing or closing the unhygienic, overcrowded urban cowsheds and controlling adulteration or accidental contamination. Tuberculous cattle were potentially deadly, befouling the milk at source, particularly as it passed through ulcerated udders. A gross example was obvious—the 'veritable living skeleton'—as were heavily infected carcasses of beef cattle after slaughter.[7] It was more difficult to detect those with hidden infections. Enter tuberculin, Koch's failed cure, which was to enjoy a series of unintended afterlives, thanks to its immunological role. With the use of tuberculin, even quality herds kept in pristine conditions—attention-grabbing examples included Queen Victoria's at Home Farm, Windsor and that of the Massachusetts Agricultural College—were shown to be carriers in the 1890s.

Tuberculin became the technical solution to the cattle cleanup campaigns waged at the end of the 19th and for much of the 20th century. It originally involved administering a small dose of tuberculin under a cow's skin and taking the temperature some hours after the injection—a rise in temperature indicated a positive reaction. The same basic immunological reaction had caused the severe temperature spikes and fever after Koch's therapeutic injections as the tuberculin reacted with the primed immune system of the host.

Tuberculin testing wasn't infallible. The early techniques needed refining. Repeated use highlighted practical problems— farmers found it disturbed their cows and the milking routine— and the number of false positives and negatives had to be minimized. In Britain, in the interwar period the Medical Research Council included tuberculin tests as part of its tuber-culosis remit to ensure purity and potency of the testing prod-uct. This had shown alarming variability. Tuberculin testing of cattle required the political will to make it work effectively and farmers had to be convinced that testing was worth the disrup-tion and financial hit. Funds had to be found to compensate those whose livelihoods would otherwise be destroyed along with their diseased cattle. Compensation had to be paid at a strategic point. If the same amount could be claimed for an older, heavily diseased animal that had yielded an income through its contaminated milk and for a young, barely infected one, there was little incentive to test early. Different countries developed their own programmes for using tuberculin. The Danish government accepted the advice of its leading veterinar-ian Bernhard Bang (1848–1932). He adapted the 'stamping out' policy developed against cattle plague. Cattle were to be tested early. Reactors were separated so as not to contaminate the clean herd, which could be used to breed. Advanced cases were slaughtered immediately with compensation, and the isolated slight cases fattened for meat. This was copied with modifica-tions in many countries; Germany, for instance, placed greater reliance on breeding disease-free herds.

Ironically Koch stalled and in some European cities over-turned nascent efforts to control the tubercle bacillus in the food chain after he declared in 1901 that bovine tuberculosis was of little consequence as a source of human disease. Such was his influence that various commissions were set up in the first decade of the 20th century to be sure that he was right. Their reports revealed how complicated the bacteriology was and differences of opinion rested in part on what questions scientists and clinicians asked of the bacilli and their human and animal hosts. The consensus swung away from Koch, who modified his own views. The international veterinary congress in Rome in 1912 issued new guidelines for inspection of cattle. Veterinarians tended to be less cluttered in their thinking about the absolute role of bacteria in causing bovine disease. They were keen to gain the professional advancement that leadership in a public health issue could bring. Anti-tuberculosis campaigners taxed governments with implementing measures to reduce the threat from infected milk but the outbreak of the First World War stalled many good intentions and made enforcement difficult.

When active campaigns could begin again, tuberculin testing was to the fore. Late entry into the war, less devastation on the ground, a greater will during the Progressive Era? It was the USA that led the way. Starting in 1917 the Bureau of Animal Industry, a federal agency, set out to test all cattle with tuberculin. All 'reactors'—cows that showed a positive response—were slaughtered and the farmer compensated. By 1940, 300 million cattle had been tested and four million reactors destroyed. Only two counties in California had more than the acceptable level of reactors—set at half a per cent of the total number of milk cows. In Britain it was not until the 1960s that a similarly broad scheme was put into place and properly funded. Instead licences were offered in the 1920s for various grades of milk, which reflected levels of testing, inspection, and pasteurization. At the top,

'Certified' and 'Grade A (tuberculin-tested)' herds were expected to bring a premium price for their milk. Theoretically consumers would pay for the best milk and the farmer would therefore want to go to the bother of testing and maintaining a tuberculosis-free herd. The economic reality of the depression years meant that even the small supply of tuberculin-tested milk exceeded demand. Aside from the laissez-faire market-force-driven approach was the belief among some tuberculosis specialists that exposure to the tubercle bacillus in milk would act as a natural inoculant, helping to protect rather than harm children.

Pasteurization posed a conundrum. Heat-treating did indeed render milk safe by killing the tubercle bacilli (and other germ contaminants) and was therefore a successful public health measure, even if it did affect the taste and the nutritional value. It did nothing to address the underlying problems of poor animal husbandry and poor post-cow handling before pasteurizing. Yet it was another prong of the aggressive stance in some American states and cities, Massachusetts (1910), Chicago (1908), and New York (1912). The incidence of non-pulmonary tuberculosis fell by nearly two-thirds in New York City between 1910 and 1925. How much of this decline could be attributed to pasteurization alone is difficult to tell given the range of other measures in a city with an aggressive tuberculosis control policy. Pasteurization became widespread across America in the 1920s. France essentially became a country of compulsory pasteurization in 1935, Sweden in 1937. Britain followed belatedly in 1960.

Never Mind the Calf

What worked for cattle also worked for children (and adults). The Viennese paediatrician Clemens von Pirquet (1874–1929) was the first to exploit the diagnostic properties of tuberculin systematically. The procedure was simple: a scrubbed forearm, two quick scratches with a needle, a drop of tuberculin on each scratch, wait for 48 hours to check the outcome. A positive was a measureable inflamed area of at least 5 mm diameter at one or both contact sites. The results of von Pirquet's trial among 1,400 clinically disease-free children under 14 years of age revealed that more than 80 per cent gave positive reactions. Some argued that this showed the development of a full-blown immunity to the disease. Something had to explain why, with near-universal levels of exposure—measured by tuberculin tests and adult autopsy records of those who had died of other causes but showed healed tuberculous lesions—only about 10 per cent developed the disease. Not everyone agreed that immunity had been achieved. They suggested instead that a positive test result merely showed sufficient exposure to the bacillus for the immune system to produce antibodies able to react with the fresh antigenic proteins in the tuberculin. The meaning of the test would prove a trickier problem to solve than its mechanics. Various different tuberculin tests were developed. Charles Mantoux (1877–1947) injected deeper into the skin and Albert Calmette (1866–1933) dropped tuberculin into the eyes.

. Von Pirquet's research was part of his wider interests in allergy. He coined the term from the Greek *allos* ('other') and *ergon* ('work or action'). Similarly Calmette's eye drop test was part of his wider interests in immunology, bacteriology, and toxicology. In French Indochina he had tried Koch's tuberculin as a cure for tuberculosis and leprosy with dreadful results, but he remained interested in its potential as a preventive measure after his return to France. In 1908, in conjunction with the veterinarian and fellow Pasteurian Camille Guérin (1872–1961), Calmette had a breakthough.

Their attempts to attenuate the bovine tubercle bacillus in a similar manner to Pasteur's classic experiments with rabies had been dogged by culturing difficulties. The addition of ox bile to their culture medium did the trick. By 1913 successive rounds of the three-weekly subculturing procedure had produced a sufficiently weakened strain of the bacillus for experimental inoculation of cattle. While they waited to determine the protective effect war broke out with Germany. Lille was taken in the autumn of 1914 and the precious cattle requisitioned by the Germany army. Calmette clandestinely conducted autopsies and found no evidence of disease, but the conditions were hardly conducive to concrete proof of the vaccine's efficacy.

After the end of the war Calmette and Guérin moved to Paris and work continued. By this time the strain of the bacillus had undergone undefined genetic changes, noticeable in its appearance as well as its reduced virulence. The first human test of the BCG—Bacillus Calmette-Guérin—vaccine took place in 1921 when a baby whose tuberculous mother had died immediately after giving birth was given an oral dose of the vaccine at three, five, and seven days of age. The child was housed with the grandmother, whose sputum contained tubercle bacilli: the kind of living conditions the L'Oeuvre Grancher had wanted to avoid. A clinical examination at six months revealed no signs of tuberculosis. A von Pirquet test (or other similar one) could not be used. The preventive inoculation had already triggered the body's immunological reaction just as if the child had been infected with the disease from its grandmother or any other source. This side effect of vaccination in people and cattle would be a sticking point in the future.

9. A fund-raising poster for the French national anti-tuberculosis association featuring Albert Calmette as the 'saviour' of children. He co-developed the BCG vaccine against tuberculosis, a specific measure most widely adopted in France before the Second World War. (*Wellcome Library, London*)

After this initial test, Calmette went on to vaccinate his own grandchildren and a steadily increasing number of babies at the l'Hôpital de la Charité, Paris. By 1928, 116,000 children had apparently been vaccinated with good results. Calmette was an imprecise record-keeper and an understandably enthusiastic advocate, who was perhaps too eager to report positive results. Outside of France the take-up was patchy. French-speaking Quebec in Canada adopted the procedure in 1928, but elsewhere in Canada Anglo-Saxon scepticism prevailed. Germany began a limited number of vaccinations in 1925. The rising Nazi party used it as a means of attacking the struggling Weimar government. They called a halt to this use of French science in 1931 after an accidentally contaminated batch of vaccine caused the death of seventy-one children in Lübeck, on Germany's Baltic coast. Despite careful work to show that the cause of death had been a laboratory error—contamination with an unattenuated human strain of the bacillus—the mud stuck.

The Scandinavian countries actively embraced the BCG vaccination as part of their ideals of scientific philanthropy and a nascent welfare state. In the interwar years, in the absence of mandatory vaccination there were a few small-scale trials of a sort. Those who were tuberculin-negative but didn't wish to be vaccinated acted as a control group, against which those who had accepted vaccination could be compared. Among Norwegian trainee nurses at a hospital in Oslo the non-vaccinated group showed six times the morbidity and seven times the mortality of the vaccinated group. Similar results were reported for school-age girls after a serious outbreak of tuberculosis was traced to a sick teacher. In 1927 in Gothenburg, Sweden, Arvid Wallgren, professor of paediatrics, began offering BCG to the family members of a confirmed tuberculosis patient and to all subsequent children born to those families. By 1933 he was claiming positive results as the number of child deaths in these high-risk families declined.

Sweden, Denmark, and Norway launched vigorous campaigns to vaccinate increasingly large sectors of their tuberculin-negative population. It made sense to target those who might, by their work, spread the disease. So, Sweden legislated to offer vaccination to schoolteachers and their pupils in 1944, with an extremely high take-up rate. It was made mandatory for staff in state mental hospitals and the dental service and among trainee nurses and medical students. In 1947 Norway made vaccination with BCG compulsory for its tuberculin-negative population as a means of dealing with the increased incidence of the disease after the ravages of the Second World War. It followed up this national programme by joining its Scandinavian neighbours in founding the International Tuberculosis Campaign, or Joint Enterprise. Working in concert with the newly founded United Nations International Children's Emergency Fund (UNICEF), this programme offered help with mass vaccination wherever a country in Europe was minded to vaccinate its young population and needed help to achieve this goal. Based on its own experience and commitment, the Joint Enterprise was quite clear that for BCG to be effective it must be used as widely as possible. They were not interested in helping with partial programmes. The coverage in Europe was impressive—Austria, Czechoslovakia, Finland, Greece, Yugoslavia, Hungary, Poland, and Italy all signed up. Germany had already benefited from a unilateral Danish project. Opinions were still divided, however, and when Italian doctors opposed vaccination Italy withdrew in 1950. By this time the programme's reach had spread beyond Europe to North Africa, the Middle East, the

Indian subcontinent and Sri Lanka, Ecuador, and Mexico. Japan also began an extensive programme, with universal vaccination of infants in 1951 followed by revaccination of school-age children beginning in 1954. BCG was produced locally at various locations and over time different strains were evolving, although the implication of this was not realized until later. Nor was it understood that different strains of *Mycobacterium tuberculosis* had variable effects on people in different regions of the globe, which rendered the vaccination less protective.

Britain (including its white colonies) had largely turned away from BCG. In the 1920s the MRC developed a couple of vaccines but these gave poor results, clouding belief in the potential of prevention through inoculation. The statisticians at the London School of Hygiene and Tropical Medicine, Britain's premier institute for epidemiology, considered that the continental trials could not be judged to have given unequivocal results; there were too many methodological flaws. Britain appeared to be committed to sanatoria—there were 40,000 beds by 1938—but the lethargy was in part a wider one, which saw a poor take-up for diphtheria vaccination too. Where immunity could be improved this was best done through the time-honoured regime of general strengthening of the body. Since the tuberculosis rates were falling, this and the other measures—dispensaries, provision for acute hospital beds—must be working.

Some argued that vaccination, like the pasteurization of milk, plastered over the cracks of underlying problems. This could refer to the distressing conditions in which the poor were obliged to live, especially in urban areas during the hungry thirties. Others thought it would encourage the youth of the nation to revert to the kind of slovenly living that had weakened the resistance of their parents and grandparents to the germ, counteracting the healthy living propaganda that issued forth from anti-tuberculosis campaigners. Only slowly in a socialist-led postwar Britain was BCG offered to nurses (partly to counter the extreme shortage of sanatorium staff), medical students, and contacts of tuberculosis patients who did not yet show a positive tuberculin test. In the 1950s school-leavers were generally offered the vaccine and a large trail of 50,000 schoolchildren gave convincing results after a ten-year follow-up in 1963 so that the scheme was extended beyond the trial. Scotland had already instigated testing and vaccination programmes.

America held out against BCG. Fears over virulence were heightened by culture experiments at the laboratory attached to Trudeau's Saranac Lake sanatorium in the 1920s. Alternative home-grown vaccines using dead rather than attenuated living strains were researched with Rockefeller money at the Henry Phipps Institute at the University of Pennsylvania, Philadelphia in the 1930s. After tests in rabbits, clinical trials were organized in Jamaica. The island was recognized to be firmly in the disease's grip. Initially inmates in a mental hospital were used as experimental subjects, but when the numbers of tuberculin negatives ran low—institutions of this sort tended to have a high percentage of tuberculous sufferers—the numbers were made up from the general population in Kingston. The locals were understandably annoyed at being experimented on when they had expected care. This feeling was borne out by the vaccine trials' failure, which showed little difference between the 11,000 vaccinated and non-vaccinated controls.

In an extended trial that began in 1935 another marginal group—members of various tribes of Native Americans—was used for a further assessment of BCG. Results issued in 1946 listed six deaths among the 1,500 or so vaccinated and 53 among the same number of unvaccinated. One of the trial's authors J. D. Aronson ran a further randomized trial vaccinating newborns on Native American reservations, which he again interpreted favourably. In what could be seen as a similar study among urban infants in New York, William Hallock Park, head of the city's laboratories, concluded that it was better 'as a public health measure' to extract children from tuberculous homes rather than waste resources on BCG which did not provide protection.[8]

Aronson became a very lonely advocate of BCG in the United States, a position that, unlike Britain's, did not change after the Second World War. The USA remained wedded to the view that BCG 'may lead to a false sense of security which could result in failure to observe precautions that would otherwise be taken'.[9] Health was a matter of individual responsibility. Tuberculosis control and social control shared much common ground. Lurking in the background were racial susceptibilities, which the rise of germ theory had only partially put to one side.

Racial Hygiene

Thinking on racial susceptibilities had significant and often unpleasant undertones. It helped dictate how vulnerable groups were treated as the extent of their tuberculosis infection was acknowledged and fed into ideas of racial superiority and inferiority. A priori assumptions as to which races were particularly susceptible or immune to tuberculosis remained powerful if fluid as immunology and epidemiology developed in the first half of the 20th century. Might resistance to the disease be a trait that some races had? Yes, possibly, depending on when, where, and why the question was asked.

Immigrant Polish Jews in America's inner cities in the 1900s had a tuberculosis mortality rate of 170 per 100,000 of the population. This compared favourably with a tuberculosis death rate of 210 per 100,000 for whites born in America. Irish-born immigrants fared much worse, with rates ranging from 400 to 600 per 100,000. The Jews did better, it was argued, because they were habituated to city living—having been forced into ghettos for centuries—where they had built up a racial immunity to the disease, and because of their dietary practices. As new immigrants they were not invulnerable; it was a relative not an absolute scale, but they were apparently less vulnerable than others. Early American public health campaigns stressed the positive aspects of the way Jews chose to live. They wanted to use them as an example to others. Later, when they had lived longer in the slums of America's cities, environmental pressures would overtake the supposed 'biological racial peculiarity'.[10] Jews would then find themselves targeted for exclusion from entering America like anyone else who failed to meet the eugenicists' criteria.

In Europe the Prague-born, German-speaking ethnic Jew and novelist Franz Kafka (1883–1924) would try to escape the racial tag of tuberculosis for as long as he could. Once he accepted the diagnosis of pulmonary and laryngeal tuberculosis that would kill him, rather than the weak heart he had hoped was his trouble, he also acknowledged that he could not escape his ethnic identity. Kafka did not wish to see his body and then his illness as marked by the traits that others attributed to the Jewish race. For ironically, both within and without the Jewish community, Jews were thought by some in the first half of the 20th century to be still marked by the characteristic body shape of the *habitus phthisicus*. The Greek idea of a particular body shape was still doing the rounds after two thousand years. Kafka referred to his body as 'too long for its weakness'.[11] Cultural Zionism and the German Jewish gymnastics movements would try to counter such pessimism in the face of the insurmountable 'final solution'.

In Germany tuberculosis was described as a 'racial poison'. Although Germany was in the forefront of health insurance, public sanatoria, and open-air schools, there were some who criticized such welfare policies for keeping the 'unfit' alive. German eugenicists regarded the tubercle bacillus as 'the friend of the race', such was its power to weed out the unfit members of society. They regarded sanatoria not so much as places of cure, but as somewhere to segregate the sick compassionately and to stop the dilution of the race by preventing them from reproducing. There were calls to constrain the free marriage of those suffering from any of the unholy triumvirate of tuberculosis, sexually transmitted diseases, and inherited mental illnesses. Active programmes of hereditarian medicine called for better population data, and for this to be correlated with medical records, enlarging upon the kinds of family studies of tuberculosis by the British eugenicist Karl Pearson.

During the First World War, as civilians suffered from shortages of food and fuel, the hand of the eugenicists was strengthened. Their role in anti-tuberculosis organizations increasingly received official endorsement as the state took on a more direct role in welfare provision. At the same time the incidence of tuberculosis and the number of deaths increased and continued to do so in the immediate aftermath of the war and the worldwide influenza pandemic. When the French took control of the industrial Rhineland, under a League of Nations edict, their troops were accused of spreading tuberculosis among the occupied German population to deliberately dilute the strength of the race.

As Germany struggled in the interwar years the racial hygiene societies pressed for greater attempts at tuberculosis control. There were calls for better research into the relationship between heredity and disease, the use of marriage certificates that indicated fitness for reproduction, sterilization of the unfit, and the screening of workers to ensure the best biological types were employed in areas of national worth. The up and coming Nazi Party reminded the populace how much it spent on the institutional care of the sick. While there was a greater emphasis on the mentally ill, disabled, and those they deemed socially undesirable, the time would come for the tuberculous too. Ideology hardened into inflexible laws in the 1930s after the Nazis came to power. Forced sterilization was legalized and prohibitive marriage laws, dominated by their focus on separating the Jewish and Aryan races, included the tuberculous in their remit. The disease was an explicit problem of heredity and subject to the new rules of racial hygiene.

As the death rate from the chronic form of the disease fell, detection by X-ray of early latent cases among the German youth became a new priority. Within the tuberculous sanatoria the Nazi doctor Kurt Heissmeyer recommended in 1943 the sorting of patients by 'racial value' as well as 'organic condition' when deciding if they were worth treating. At the Neuengamme concentration camp he used Jewish children and adults for his experiments on the immunity to tuberculosis, and not just because of their easy availability: in his view their racial inferiority made them particularly easy subjects to infect and in which to monitor the progress of the disease. When medical murder was approved—'a pilot scheme for the holocaust'—the

T4 euthanasia programme began its 'coercion, control and kill-ing'.[12] Concentration camp populations were reduced as the sick were liquidated. T4 was superseded by the Aktion 14f13 initiative, which stepped up the killing machine on its the way to the 'final solution'. Under this plan the SS used mobile X-ray machines to diagnose the tuberculosis of an estimated 100,000 people in occupied Poland and the Soviet Union. All were shot.

The 'Disease of Civilization'

The Nazi racial excesses were unique but they intersected with two key concepts—'virgin soil' and 'tubercularization'—which shaped attitudes and policies elsewhere. The idea of 'virgin soil' initially referred to non-immune races and accounted for their devastating experiences with tuberculosis. Native Americans, it was thought, had not had any experience of tuberculosis until contact with white settlers. Moreover their outdoor lifestyle was attuned to preventing the disease. Once exposed to the white man and his germs, they swiftly succumbed to the disease. Herded onto reservations, living in insanitary conditions (for which they were blamed), encouraged to engage in static agriculture rather than hunting, as part of the 'civilizing process', Native Americans had to contend with many infectious diseases, including tuberculosis. Death rates ran at about 3,000 per 100,000 of the population each year in the early 20th century (the statistics were poorly kept). At least on the reservation they were not much of a focus of infection.

Such an understanding of virgin soil invited an apathetic response towards the sick. It was the same initially with tuberculous black Americans, as they left the rural south for northern cities. Frederick Hoffman, chief statistician at the Prudential

Insurance Company based in Newark, New Jersey, confidently declared early in the 20th century that such was the severity of the disease among this race that natural selection would run its course and the race die out. The Prudential avoided taking on black customers. Black migrant workers in South Africa's Rand gold-mines were also sent to their 'healthy' homes on the veldt once their disease was manifest. Racial inferiority rather than the appalling working and living conditions they encountered were blamed.

In the 1910s the meaning of 'virgin soil' was modified. It was no longer so much an innate property of the body, something 'fixed in the blood', that helped certain races defend themselves against the disease. Now the emphasis was on a much more quickly acquired immunity, more Lamarckian than Darwinian. Members of any race could achieve acquired immunity, given the right exposure to the bacillus, in the right conditions. An artificially induced acquired immunity was thought to under-pin the auto-intoxication associated with graduated labour for instance. It also applied subsequently to the vaccination with BCG. Naturally occurring acquired immunity was the result of a gradual 'tubercularization': the routine exposure to the right amount of the tubercle bacillus as part of daily life. Tuberculari-zation would sensitize but not mount an outright assault on the body, allowing it to resist later larger exposures without devel-oping the disease. This was the case for the majority of white Europeans and North Americans. Their bodies safely contained the bacillus in healed primary lesions. They had no symptoms and died of something else. Taken to its extreme, ridding the population of all exposure might be counter-productive as there would be no natural tubercularization, but at the time this was a problem for the future.

The concern for the previously unexposed was to ensure that their tubercularization was carefully managed. This allowed for a little more optimism, reported Lyle Cummins (1873–1949), one of the field's leading voices. Cummins repeated the mantra that tuberculosis was a disease of civilization. If the process of 'civilization' was managed appropriately, there was no reason those populations experiencing tuberculosis for the first time, in the wake of European colonization of the tropics for example, could not be spared the excess tubercular mortality they were suffering. This, Cummins argued, might mean that the 'civilizing mission' would be slowed down, keeping the native population out of unhealthy urban areas unless they were working there and sending them home to healthful conditions if they became ill to recuperate.

Cummins's long engagement with tuberculosis was conducted during a career with stints in Egypt in the Royal Army Medical Corps, in London at the Royal Army Medical College's vaccine department, and in France as an army pathologist during the First World War. After the war he was made tuberculosis professor at the Welsh National School of Medicine in Cardiff, where he investigated links between this and other mining diseases. He was seconded in the later 1920s to advise on tuberculosis in South African mines. Cummins's work on the Rand led him to change his immunological theories again.

In his 'modified virgin soil' theory he returned to reliance upon racial differences. He thought that Africans exhibited a 'real inborn lack of power to develop...resistance' and a 'biological dissimilarity in the average response to tuberculous infection'.[13] This dissimilarity, fed by pathological studies of tubercle lesions in different races, was evidence of an intermediate stage between virgin soil, but before full tubercularization.

In this fluid phase tubercularization was sufficient to prevent the fulminating disease but insufficient to prevent a breakdown under hard living and working conditions. Cummins believed that African miners, who faced a potentially lethal combination of silicosis, pneumonia, and tuberculosis, were indeed showing this transitional response to the disease.

Cummins's new ideas, more fatalistic than his earlier ones on tubercularization, helped condemn the mine workers and black South Africans more generally and fed into the prejudices of the apartheid state after the Second World War. On a time-scale measured in several generations, improving conditions in the mines and townships would achieve only so much, so why bother in the short term? There were lots of potential miners and vast sums of money to be made from minerals. The best plan was continued segregation, which sought to keep the miners in labour camps and the general population away from urban areas unless they were required to work there, in which case they must be isolated in townships.

The immunological picture was continually jumbled. The boundaries between individuals and groups, races and ethnicities, were frequently blurred and the data on which conclusions were drawn can be seen with hindsight to lack statistical rigour. Such fractious differences initially faded in the wake of the discovery of antibiotics. This was to transform the image of tuberculosis from blight of youth and racial poison to a curable condition.

VIII

⤛⤜

STREPTOMYCIN & CO.

Something from the Soil

B anner headlines announced the arrival of first one and then a combination of drugs that could cure tuberculosis. It had after all only been some two thousand-plus years in the offing. Each generation of doctors and patients longed for the seemingly impossible. In the early years streptomycin and its successors would mop up a disease on the wane in the developing world and hold out great hope for an improvement elsewhere as health became a global prerogative after the Second World War. The public health programmes that targeted tuberculosis were strengthened by innovations in X-ray technology that helped diagnosis, aiming to catch the disease in a pincer movement. The future appeared to be rosy, the blush of health replacing the hot, hectic flush.

Antibiotics seem miraculous. Chemicals produced by micro-organisms, antibiotics can inhibit the growth of or kill other micro-organisms—including disease-causing bacteria. Most usefully, many can do this from inside our bodies with only minimal harm to us. Harnessing the potential of 'bacterial antagonism' had been a goal of the early proponents of germ theory. Louis Pasteur described it in 1877 as 'perhaps the greatest hopes for therapeutics'.[1]

The first and most famous antibiotic that could be used in humans was penicillin. Penicillin is effective against what are termed the gram-positive bacteria. When they are stained using a technique named after its inventor, Hans Gram, they appear under the microscope as dark blue or violet rods or blobs. Streptomycin followed hard on the heels of penicillin. It has a different spectrum of activity and is used against gram-negative bacteria (which show as red or pink when counter-stained), including the plague bacillus. It is also effective against acid-fast bacteria (those that resist being decoloured by acids during staining), such as the *Mycobacterium tuberculosis*. The discovery of streptomycin would bring the biochemist and microbiologist Selman Waksman (1888–1973) a Nobel Prize in 1952: the second for tuberculosis. It remains a matter of debate whether this honour should have been shared with members of Waksman's team, in particular Albert Schatz (1922–2005), who successfully sued for a share of the patent royalties.

Waksman, a Russian-born American, had spent his research career at what would become a part of Rutgers University. When it was still the Agricultural Experiment Station at New Brunswick, Waksman began his pursuit of the microbiology of soil. Many soil microbes live by digesting the remains of plant and animal bodies or by preying upon each other. Waksman was fired by how they differ in specific ecological niches—soils, bogs, and peat beds—and how they contributed to healthy, productive soil. He worked closely with 'ray fungi' or the actinomycetes. These bacteria, named for their production of thread-like filaments, give fresh, moist soil its characteristic

earthy scent, beloved of gardeners as they dig. Some actinomycetes—including the *Streptomyces*—interested Waksman because
of their inhibitory effects on the growth of other soil micro-
organisms, but they were only one of many micro-organisms
and this effect was one of many such interactions. Streptomycin
would later be produced from certain strains of a species of this
subgroup, *Streptomyces griseus*.

It seems a perfectly obvious trajectory: soil-bacteria specialist
'sees' an antagonistic effect between bacteria in the laboratory,
isolates the organism, and then makes a biologically active
extract; tests are run in animals and humans; a life-saving drug
results. Can you miss something if you are not looking for it? As
in the penicillin story there were more twists, turns, and perhaps
opportunities passed up. In 1915 Waksman noticed that there
was an inverse relationship between concentrations of actinomycetes and other bacteria in a soil sample. In 1916 he isolated
Streptomyces griseus (known as *Actinomycetes griseus*, until Waksman and a colleague reclassified it in 1943) and described some of
its properties but didn't test it as an 'antibiotic'. In 1932 Waksman, as a soil expert, accepted a grant from the leading American research and tuberculosis associations to consider the
longevity of the tubercle bacillus in the soil and the role of soil
bacteria in their demise. Pasteur had argued that the soil must be
antagonistic to pathological bacteria; otherwise it would hold an
ever-increasing melange of germs. Waksman asked a student to
conduct the research; the latter did a thorough job, but neither
wanted to continue with the tuberculosis-related work. In 1935
Waksman did not pursue an interesting-looking test-tube containing a culture of bird tubercle bacilli, killed by a contaminat-
ing mould. His interests and successes remained elsewhere. In
1939 priorities changed.

Waksman was well placed to reorient his gaze. Inspiration came in part from the work of Oswald Avery and his former graduate student René Dubos. Dubos and Avery developed a culture method to compel one kind of bacteria to feed on another in a highly specific way. This contrived bacterial antagonism relied upon an enzyme to strip away the otherwise impenetrable protective coat of a pneumonia germ. Without its coat, phagocytes—defence cells of the immune system—could engulf and destroy the naked germs. In 1939 Dubos prepared a solution containing the active chemical produced by another antagonistic bacteria, *Bacillus brevis*. Tests in mice (slightly antedating similar experiments with penicillin) showed that this solution could be used as an antibiotic rather than the whole organism. Principles and techniques: antibiotics from soil organisms had become tangible.

Waksman was working on micro-organisms and fermentation with money from the chemical giant Merck & Co., about twenty miles up the road from his laboratory. In 1939 they backed him to search for soil micro-organisms with antibiotic potential. In an academic–industrial synergy Waksman was to direct the microbiology, while Merck assumed responsibility for the chemistry, pharmacology, and animal and clinical trials. Merck would own the research results, take out all necessary patents, and pay a royalty to Rutgers as the host university. When the realization of streptomycin's potential to cure disease and yield enormous profit hit, Waksman and George Merck changed the rules. The Rutgers Research and Endowment fund were given the patent and Merck gave up exclusive rights to develop and market the drug. Waksman's strategic soil-screening programme was initially a small exploratory one, among the other projects running in his department. Then according to his assistant, the chemist Boyd Woodruff, he strode into the laboratory after learning more about the progress with penicillin in Florey's Oxford laboratory and said: 'drop everything. See what these Englishmen have discovered a mold can do. I know the actinomycetes will do better!'[2]

Actinomycin was the first product Waksman and his colleagues derived from the actinomycetes. Helped by the chemical and pharmacological staff at Merck, they were able to determine that although it was potently bactericidal it was too toxic in animals. The same fate befell the first of the antibiotics produced from a streptomycium. Streptothricin appeared to be well tolerated but caused delayed kidney damage. These near-misses encouraged the newly formed department of microbiology at Rutgers to take on more graduate students and expand the search. The early work also provided important lessons on technique. Waksman abandoned the complex and several-month-long soil enrichment of Dubos for a simpler and much quicker plate-cultivating technique using the familiar Petri dish. Another hopeful contender—streptomycin—was isolated in 1943 by Albert Schatz, one of Waksman's fifty-strong team. After the extract was crystallized and shown to be water-soluble, its broad range of activity was satisfactorily tested. *Mycobacterium tuberculosis* featured as an acid-fast bacillus among a list of twenty-one other gram-negative and gram-positive bacteria when the research was published in 1944 but there was no indication that this was being posited as a potential cure for tuberculosis.

Before that research paper went to press, Waksman entertained William Feldman (1892–1974) of Mayo Clinic's Institute of Experimental Medicine. Feldman, a veterinary pathologist, was already working closely with his clinical colleague Corwin

Hinshaw (1902–2001). Together they were testing some of the existing sulfa drugs in tuberculous guinea pigs and sick patients. The results of their initial animal tests with the limited amount of streptomycin that Waksman's team could produce were good enough for Merck & Co. to make the decision to pursue industrial-scale fermentation to increase output of the drug. With this in hand, a more extensive guinea pig trial in July 1944 was followed in November with a course of treatment involving advanced cases at the Mineral Springs Sanatorium. As is often the case, those with little to lose and much to gain were chosen for the experimental therapy. The first celebrations were for Patricia Thomas, who received five painful courses of the drug over six months. Each course lasted up to eighteen days and involved regular intramuscular injections. The possible side effects were giddiness, dizziness, and deafness. Having coped with these, and as her condition progressed, Thomas received further thoracic surgery before leaving the sanatorium in 1946. She married and had three children. The stuff dreams are made of for patient and doctor alike.

It was inevitable, despite Hinshaw and Feldman's moratorium on personal press appearances, that news of the miracle cure would be unstoppable and demand for streptomycin insatiable. At least six American companies committed themselves to large-scale production by 1946. Wartime experience in equitable allocation of essential products led to the Civilian Production Administration in 1945. They continued to oversee streptomycin's distribution after controls on other goods were lifted in 1947. After the early tests with seriously ill patients more systematic trials were undertaken. The drug manufacturers asked the American Trudeau Society to oversee the use of over a million dollars' worth of streptomycin among sanatorium patients. The Veterans' Administration Hospital worked with tuberculosis personnel being repatriated after the war. In both these trials everyone received the drug, according to the best-guess standard dose, which was refined as time went by. Among the armed forces personnel patients acted as their own controls. X-rays were taken at intervals to chart a patient's progress during the two-month period before streptomycin was given and the four-month treatment period. The X-rays were read blind— the doctor did not know at what stage the X-ray had been taken—but no one remained untreated. The immediate results were very encouraging.

Across the pond, the British made a virtue out of necessity. American streptomycin was expensive and foreign exchange scarce. Amid rumours about toxicity the authorities urged caution on a tuberculous public understandably pressing for the new drug. Waksman would always maintain with quiet disdain that the British had overreacted about toxicity. Facilities for home production were beginning but in the interim the British government bought a relatively small amount of the drug (50 kg) for the MRC in November 1946. A little was set aside for cases of tuberculous meningitis, where its speed of action and ability to bring children back from the brink was almost miraculous. In comparison with adult cases, children have far fewer bacteria in their bodies, which means that the chance of mutations and resistance is greatly lowered. Most of the streptomycin was used to set up a randomized clinical trial led by a team of MRC luminaries including Austin Bradford Hill (1897–1991), Philip D'Arcy Hart (1900–2006), and Marc Daniels (1917–53) and involving about a hundred patients. Half of the group received the drug while the control group received the usual sanatorium care but not the drug. Given that the drug had to be administered by intramuscular injection, it was decided that use of a placebo was not practical. When there was not enough to go around it was not considered unethical to treat some and not others; that was going to happen anyway. It has become a legend in the history of clinical trials.

Patients were carefully selected to meet definite criteria, which would prevent undue suffering. They were to have active disease in both lungs, which was to be confirmed by evidence of bacteria from their sputum. The extent of their disease would make them unsuitable for the popular alternative of collapse therapy. This way a patient who could have had thoracic surgery was not denied a chance of better health by being enrolled in the study if the drugs failed. Older chronic cases were omitted. The preferred age range was from 15 to 25 (raised later to 30). Should the treatment work, those with the most to gain would be the recipients. To prevent any local bias in who had the drug, the trial's statistical expert Bradford Hill randomized the patients—names were sent out in sealed envelopes from the MRC to the participating hospitals. Great care was taken to ensure that like was compared with like by matching drug recipients and controls for disease severity. Thus the trial could potentially provide an unbiased assessment of the effect of streptomycin on this kind of tuberculosis, notwithstanding all its vagaries of self-healing and relapse. Following multiple blind appraisals of patients' X-rays as well as sputum and body weight assessments, the MRC agreed with the Americans: pulmonary tuberculosis responded to streptomycin.

A Quick Fight Back

While the trials were under way the streptomycin supply was necessarily limited and a black market developed. If availability

was one serious problem faced by patients hoping for a streptomycin cure, the other was the rise of resistance. It became
apparent that not all the estimated ten million (10^7) to one billion (10^9) bacilli in a case of cavitary pulmonary tuberculosis in
a patient's body are identical and therefore affected by the drug
in the same way. This would later be shown to be as a consequence of random mutations as they divide and replicate. Some
of these mutations mean that they can resist the drug's action.
Such mutations happen approximately once in every million
(10^6) to ten million (10^7) replications. At this mutation rate, in
this number of bacilli in a typical case, the rise of resistance was
indeed common. Once resistance had developed additional use
of the drug had no further effect: after a temporary improvement patients would once more begin to deteriorate. The success of something from the soil would be saved by something
else from Sweden: para-aminosalicylic acid, or PAS.

PAS is derived from salicylic acid, as is that mainstay of many a
home medicine cabinet, aspirin. Its development was independent from that of streptomycin but PAS shared the new interest in
biochemical understanding of microbes and their metabolic
processes. During a series of well-thought-out experiments in
the late 1930s the biochemist Frederick Bernheim discovered that
salicylic acid stimulated the growth of tubercle bacilli by helping
them take up oxygen. Next he looked for a related compound,
one that would be taken up by the bacillus, but rather than helping it would hinder this particular metabolic pathway—one of
the chemical reactions that take place within cells. This is a process known as competitive inhibition. He had little success—the
compounds he tested were too toxic—but he published his findings and in the old-fashioned way that science used to be done,
sent a colleague, Jörgen Lehmann, an offprint of the paper.

After a peripatetic career, Lehmann had taken the post of chemical pathologist at the Sahlgrenska Hospital in Gothenburg, Sweden. Finding the time to investigate Bernheim's ideas in early 1943, he had a small pharmaceutical firm (Ferrosan) make a range of salicylic acid derivatives to his order. It turned out that PAS—the one he had thought would be most promising from its theoretical structure—was hard to make, which was perhaps why it had not been tested by Bernheim. The usual round of guinea pig experiments was followed by some therapeutic tests in a case of pulmonary tuberculosis in a young woman. In the autumn of 1944 'Sigrid' received PAS slightly before Patricia started on streptomycin in America. She too progressed sufficiently to undergo surgery and leave the sanatorium cured.

There was a delay to publication—Ferrosan were keen to ensure their patent. Even after the announcement paper in *The Lancet* in 1946, further difficulties in the production slowed the drug's progress. Then, while the Swedes tested their own drug against a placebo, the MRC ran a three-pronged trial of streptomycin, PAS, and the two drugs in combination. PAS-only patients benefited but also ran the risk of resistance. Given properly over a long period, the cocktail cured and essentially prevented resistance. The genes in the bacteria's chromosome that mutate to create resistance to each drug are not linked so the chance of any one bacteria becoming resistant to both drugs is very low—estimated to be one in 10^{14}—so long as the drugs are taken together and not sequentially. Still, the treatment wasn't easy. Combined treatment meant intramuscular injections and the neurological side effects of streptomycin along with large, frequent oral doses of PAS, which induced constant nausea (because PAS is rapidly metabolized and its breakdown products easily excreted in urine). With the cocktail idea in place the search was on for more easily administered drugs or those that could help where resistance had already been developed during treatment.

Isonicotinic acid hydrazide, usually known as isoniazid, was the best one for the job. It was cheap, highly active, relatively easy to administer by mouth, and minimally toxic for most patients, although there can be neurological and liver problems. It was cheap because it had already been synthesized in Prague in 1912 and could not be patented. Once its activity against the tubercle bacillus was agreed upon in the early 1950s companies anywhere could begin manufacture. Determining its activity was more complex, with unrelated projects in Germany, France, and America during and immediately after the war. It is a testament to what drives scientific research that such work continued even where conditions were poor, although the wartime rise of tuberculosis was a serious worry. Nevertheless the disruptive effect of war and its immediate aftermath stymied communication. There were physical and emotional barriers to be overcome, as well as the usual commercial concerns of drug companies. The now familiar press headlines told of miraculous cures as news of isoniazid treatment leaked from the Sea View Hospital—a sanatorium on Staten Island, New York—in February 1952. By the end of the year the basis for this euphoria had been confirmed by further rigorous trials.

There were some, like George Orwell, for whom the drugs came too late, some who failed to respond positively and in whom allergic reactions or toxicity prevented success. Resistance was a serious threat, but sensible prescribing would use more than one drug anyway because each acted in slightly different ways on the target bacilli. Despite these caveats there was now a potent combination therapy involving three front-line drugs for a previously incurable disease. And that really was something special.

Shadows and Spots: X-Rays for the Masses

The better the chances of curing a patient the more it behoves the finding of cases and finding them early. The early diagnosis mantra would become particularly meaningful in the new era of effective tuberculosis chemotherapy. Wilhelm Röntgen (1845–1923) was not attempting to find a new imaging device to help the fight against tuberculosis or any other disease, but his experiments in 1895 with electromagnetic radiation did just that. X-rays gradually allowed doctors to see inside the body. As X-ray and allied technologies developed, something of the disease's characteristic lesions, particularly in advanced stages, could be seen although tubercles remained indistinguishable.

The effects of the lesions had been visualized during life after the advent of stethoscopy (auscultation) and the technique of tapping the body (percussion) to determine whether its solid, hollow, and fluid-filled parts were as they should be. This method of diagnosis continued. So too did examination with a microscope of stained sputum samples to look for bacteria, their culture in the laboratory, and immunological testing with tuberculin. X-rays came to augment all these techniques. Fixed on a photographic plate and later celluloid film, X-ray pictures provided a permanent visual record in the medical file. Learning to hear the body involved training the ear to differentiate the complex symphony of crackles, clicks, and rattles. Learning to read the skiagram (from the Greek for 'shadow') or X-ray film, meant training the eye to appreciate the inner contours of the body and to make sense of the shadows and spots.

X-rays are two-dimensional representations of three-dimensional structures. What they literally show are the differing abilities of materials to absorb or reflect the beam of electrons which constitute an X-ray. On an X-ray film, healthy lungs appear dark grey to black because they are essentially full of low-density air. More solid organs such as the heart and bony ribs that frame the chest cavity show up as much whiter areas on the recording film. This is because X-rays easily penetrate air in the lungs while the denser tissue offers greater resistance, bouncing the X-rays back.

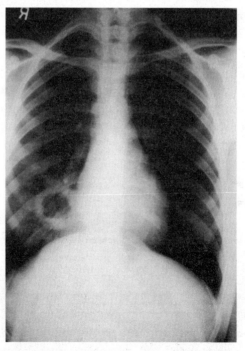

10. An X-ray of the lungs: at the base of the right lung (shown here on the left) a circular cavity is clearly visible. (*Wellcome Library, London*)

In the lung it is possible to recognize inklings of disease, which would escape notice in denser organs (tuberculosis, of course, is not the only disease that causes shadows in the lung). When something abnormal happens in the lung—like the inflammatory processes of tuberculosis—the greater quantity of blood involved, which is denser than the normal air-filled lungs, shows up by reflecting the X-rays. Thus the first trace of pulmonary tuberculosis is a faint mottling seen within the grey shadow of the lung. Well-advanced cases of disease or those replete with healed, calcified lesions are easier to read. Extensive cavities tend to speak for themselves and an abundance of calci-fied tissue was more distinct: both usually confirmed a clinical diagnosis. However, an X-ray and then a subsequent autopsy could tell quite different tales. Sanatoria, particularly expensive elite ones, soon purchased X-ray machines, bolstering their sci-entific credentials, but their catchment group had already been diagnosed. Hans Castrop and several of his fellows on the 'Magic Mountain' proudly carried their X-ray pictures around with them for ready comparison or as talismans of their inner selves. In these early years 'röntgenology' in pulmonary tuberculosis was more novelty than cutting-edge science.

During the American draft for the First World War, an urgency surrounded the sending overseas on a crowded troop ship those who could spread disease or quickly suffer a break-down during the conflict. Yet, only a few thousand men were X-rayed out of the 3.8 million examined. X-rays were expen-sive. Amassing the large number of photographic plates and skilled readers that screening involved was unrealistic, and so the procedure was restricted to problematic or disputed cases. In the interwar period, with the public sanatorium movement expanding everywhere, X-ray machines were more commonly used for assessment of admission and to monitor progress during rest and surgical cures. Dispensaries equipped with an X-ray machine could take referrals as well as offering a service to contacts of newly discovered cases. New York City's mass case-finding studies in the 1930s, which included chest X-rays of some 150,000 people, concluded that this technology was best used to diagnose those in high-risk groups: the indigent and homeless and those already corralled in prison. While interpretation of chest X-rays would continue to require specific skills, the means of producing them quickly and cheaply improved with innovations from Rio de Janeiro. In the mid-1930s Rio experienced a devastating epidemic of tuberculosis as Brazil industrialized. Manuel Dias de Abreu (1884–1962) combined a long-standing interest in improving soft tissue radiography with advances in the quality of X-ray and film equipment, including small, fast camera lenses. He developed the technique of 'abreugraphy'. This relatively inexpensive and expeditious way of taking photographs on rolls of 50 mm or 100 mm film from an X-ray image that could be displayed on a fluorescent screen would stimulate case-finding all over the world in due course. In the meantime a successful local thoracic census quickly began in Rio.

Mass miniature radiography, or MMR (the procedure was known by a variety of names in different countries), was hailed as a cost-effective means of detecting asymptomatic cases. Galvanized by the threat of tuberculosis among civilians and military personnel following the outbreak of war in 1939, MMR became part of the war effort. It sifted out those who should be referred for further follow-up, to determine the nature and extent of their lesions, active or inactive. Just as institutions had once been seen as the popular solution to a variety of problems, now the mass application of technology and ideals of industrial throughput would build aircraft and diagnose disease. Chest X-rays revealed more than tuberculosis but this was the first target.

The United States came late into the war but quickly scaled up its use of X-ray examinations. Some 20 million men were X-rayed as part of their pre-induction examination for the army and navy. By late 1942 chest X-ray had become mandatory for all recruits. The army was keen to avoid as much of the estimated $1.186 billion spent by the Veterans' Administration from 1918 to 1940 in treating service-connected tuberculosis among those in and discharged from the armed forces.[3] Mass radiography was used in factories, mines, and other institutional settings to try to ensure that production in essential industries would not be hampered.

The American Public Health Service established an Office of Tuberculosis Control to deal with the potential rise in tuberculosis cases—the first federal grant to control the disease. The office promoted X-ray screening and its funding enabled various health bureaucracies to take advantage of the war effort and encourage participation. MMR was touted as a quick, risk-free procedure that could help all. Those rejected by the military or found to be sick at work were reported to the state and municipal authorities and their contacts were checked in the normal way. A $10 billion federal budget was voted to the office for the fiscal year 1944–5 to cope with caring for the increased number of cases of tuberculosis found by screening.

In Australia the armed forces were also among the first to be screened when mass radiography began. In the civilian population the anti-tuberculosis association ran the first comprehensive industrial X-ray project in 1942 by screening the 830-strong workforce of Philips electrical industries. This was no random choice. Philips supplied replacement parts for their existing X-ray equipment and a member of staff acted as the association's honorary radiographer. Philips paid a fee of £250 for the survey. The association was grateful for the money but gained rather more in valuable experience as they reoriented their target population. From its inception in Sydney in 1910 the association had concentrated on the poor; now it aimed to screen all in a locality or a particular industry regardless of income level. Mass miniature radiography was a leveller. In 1944 the association launched a publicity drive popularizing mass X-rays. They ordered a new 35 mm camera from the USA, only to have the consignment stuck in the docks during a strike by wharf labourers. Appeals to release the equipment were successful and as part of the negotiations the union members were among the first to have a visit from the team.

Scaling Up

In postwar Europe most countries strove to restore, augment, or establish dedicated tuberculosis services and beds. Expanding facilities would help counter wartime increases or continue to drive down static or falling rates. It was hoped that excess disease would fall away as living conditions and nutrition improved in peacetime, provided cases could be identified, isolated, and if possible treated. There was a great deal of optimistic rhetoric. Tuberculosis was one of the three immediate disease priorities of the newly formed World Health Organization (the others were malaria and venereal disease). An expert committee on tuberculosis was formed in 1947 to continue the work of the United Nations Relief and Rehabilitation Administration (UNRRA) and the pre-WHO United Nations health body, the

Interim Commission. In Hungary, for instance, 6,500 pre-war beds had been reduced by early 1945, when conditions reached their worst level, to only 500. Food was extremely scarce and services in chaos. The death rate in Budapest neared 250 per 100,000. UNRRA provided such simple things as beds and blankets where needed in Europe. By 1948 the number of Hungarian sanatorium beds had increased tenfold to 5,000. An estimated 8,000 were required, however, and the goal was to set up hutments around existing hospitals in the Swedish style.

There were also attempts to rationalize overly complicated organizational structures. Previously, in France the question who would pay for which patient to enter what sanatorium had held up admissions even when a bed was available. Under the new simplified system payment for institutional care became incumbent on the *département* where the patient lived. Region-alization aimed to provide an equal distribution of beds where they were needed. French death rates rose from their pre-war level to a peak in 1941, before declining again. Paris experienced the worst of the wartime epidemic. Death rates rose from 155 deaths per 100,000 of the population in 1938 to 215 in 1941 before falling to only 72 per 100,000 in 1947. In Italy and Poland there were attempts to remove pre-war tensions between social insurance organizations and ministries of health. From a poor baseline Poland had suffered greatly. Before the war death rates in the cities were high (c.150 per 100,000) and services lim-ited—one bed for every six deaths (a frequently used compara-tive measure). By 1941 the death rate in Warsaw had risen 200 per cent. In the immediate aftermath payment for facilities and care from public funds was extremely limited but the situation began to improve as government funds for sanatorium treat-ment trickled through.

The same opportunity was taken to rationalize the provision of dispensaries, which served as the basic diagnostic unit in many countries with a tuberculosis service. These were often renamed chest clinics to tackle the continued stigma attached to tuberculosis. In Sweden the National League against Tuberculosis continued to run the dispensaries but now the money came via the government from taxation. Sweden had managed to reduce its tuberculosis death rate, despite the war, from 82 per 100,000 in 1938 to 51 per 100,000 in 1946. Charity was being replaced by statutory obligation either in recognition of the seriousness of the problem or, in some countries, because of an increased commitment to the ideals of a welfare state. Many countries followed Britain and had the state assume responsibility for the cost of institutional care for patients and social assistance for patients and dependants. France, Poland, Bulgaria, and Czechoslovakia all voted to offer a financial aid package for the tuberculous to help keep their families afloat while patients were isolated in sanatoria.

Passing legislation was the easiest part. Marc Daniels of the MRC worked for UNRRA in Italy, Poland, Czechoslovakia, Austria, and Geneva as a tuberculosis consultant and reported in 1949 on the loss of skilled doctors and nurses, and the degradation of buildings and the civilian population: 'It was not rare to find hospitals where patients had to bring their own linen if they were to have any, and no drugs were provided; frantic relatives would spend much time trying to buy such drugs as calcium gluconate on the black market, to say nothing of penicillin and, later, streptomycin.' Even in Britain, 'we are not without so-called sanatoria which have no diagnostic equipment, no facilities for active treatment, and no staff qualified to apply it if they had it, and whose patients are sent many miles away on the rare occasions when an X-ray film is thought necessary'.[4]

If this sounded bleak, Daniels was optimistic that in the wake of the war a renewed sense of national and international responsibilities would lead to a continued fall in the numbers suffering from tuberculosis. The Nordic countries had spearheaded BCG. WHO demonstration teams were already active in Greece and Poland in Europe and in China and India in Asia. The International Union against Tuberculosis (founded in 1920) retained its independence from WHO but provided an important 'forum for discussing the scientific and medico-social problems that needed to be solved in order to facilitate action planning in the fight against tuberculosis'.[5] Later The Union established a series of regional committees covering the globe and urged WHO to press for concerted action. In the meantime Daniels was aware that the death rates he quoted had not been gathered in ideal circumstances. Morbidity statistics in terms of new cases notified or discovered were even more problematic and he endorsed WHO's commitment to expanding such studies globally using tuberculin testing and, where the facilities were ready to hand, MMR. It would be a while before people realized that developing countries could not simply copy the programmes of their better-off neighbours, with expensive case-finding by X-ray and reliance upon in-patient treatment, but there was at least some enthusiasm to try and thereby acknowledge the problem.

Mass X-ray moved into a new gear in the developed world when, in addition to the static machines being set up in chest clinics, hospitals, and sanatoriums the machines were taken out into the community. In an era of mobile mass radiography the potential for targeted and whole community screening greatly increased. In 1947 the Australians were using a converted single-decker Sydney bus with space for a consulting room, photographic dark room, and storage for delicate X-ray equipment during transit to suburban and then rural areas. Upon arrival it would set up shop in an easily located building—a department store, cinema, or community centre with a good electricity supply. The X-ray equipment had to be taken off the bus and assembled and changing rooms set up, as patients were required to undress partially. Timed slots for men and women allowed for modesty between the sexes, which was important when participants were being invited to come forward voluntarily. A successful screening programme required a good take-up to be worthwhile—local community groups were asked to help with the turnout. A charge of 5 shillings per person was commuted to 10 shillings for a family of any size. X-raying the whole family in one visit typified the intended comprehensiveness of such programmes. In 1948 the Australian commonwealth and state governments jointly sponsored an anti-tuberculosis campaign that included compulsory but free X-ray screening for everyone aged 16 and over. Some herculean efforts were made to survey area populations. St Louis county, Minnesota X-rayed its entire population of 34,000 residents. Floating clinics on ships, railroad trucks, airplanes, and dog sleds were used to reach the native Alaskan people in a number of surveys beginning in 1945. By 1957 the death rate there had reached 116 per 100,000, down from an appalling 655/100,000 in 1950.

In postwar Britain the newly founded National Health Service (1946) expanded voluntary mass civilian X-ray screening using furniture vans to move the equipment around. In 1949 a fleet of self-contained units came into operation. Now the X-rays could be both taken and developed in the van, although there was still no space for the clerk who sat outside as the

X-rays were taken. The equipment came with its own power supply by towing a generator. Mindful of postwar austerity, which stymied many good intentions, some of the generators were Air Ministry surplus, left over from mobile radar units.

By the mid-1950s, mass X-ray units were using mirror cameras with a higher resolving power—the degree to which an imaging device sees as distinct and therefore records clearly the bits and pieces that make up the object under view. Larger-format film—70 or 100 mm—offered improved viewing. It was also no longer necessary to undress partially. Providing that the target population had received the message and were willing to come forward, this equipment could photograph between 600 and 700 pairs of lungs a day. Technically the programme was sound enough. For both fixed and mobile units the sticking point would turn out to be participation rates and then over time a diminishing return for the effort and expenditure.

At the end of 1945 some 797,000 civilians had been X-rayed in England and Wales. These examinations had yielded 2,900 cases of active tuberculosis. Put another way, MMR had detected an incidence of 3.6 per 1,000 of the population X-rayed. These detection rates became commonly cited figures in the tuberculosis community. They could be compared over time or from place to place. The figures could be broken down by age group or gender, and any differences tested for statistical significance. All this had been possible before, except the numbers were smaller and the time-frame to produce the statistics was much longer.

Mass X-ray facilitated an important shift towards targeting populations rather than individuals plus their immediate contacts. This had been the predominant pattern in the past with notification schemes. It provided a means of targeting health expenditure on tuberculosis where it was most needed—so long as there were adequate existing services and it was not done at the cost of 'more fundamental work in tuberculosis control'.[6] It offered the potential to pick out from the crowd those who needed treatment and who posed a threat, not just to their family, but also to their wider contacts. Crowds often meant schools, prisons, mental hospitals, or factories. Annual surveys of students and teaching staff were initiated in France, but such regularity was not always deemed necessary. Each X-ray was a radiation exposure for the subject and had a real cost regardless of who paid. This might have been as low as a shilling, the cost of a packet of twenty Woodbine cigarettes in 1944, but as incidence rates fell it became more expensive.[7]

Surveys in Britain's industrial Midlands, in the factories and steelworks of Northamptonshire, revealed both how the incidence of the disease was declining and how mass radiography could be tailored. It turned out to be much more useful in the stable population working in the boot and shoe factories than in the more mobile population of steel workers. At the shoe factory the fall to what seemed to be a standard baseline of new cases (1.23/1,000) had been achieved because after identification there had been a 'weeding out of elderly chronic cases of pulmonary tuberculosis' from the closed factory workrooms.[8] Almost half the newly discovered cases in the first survey were in males over the age of 35, many of whom had bacilli in their sputum and were deemed to have been a source of infection for some time. Women seemed to benefit too from the aftermath of the surveys. Taken together, the footwear and clothing industries, where far more women worked, gave a similar declining incidence rate for women as for men. What was different was the age group in which these rates were peaking. While tuberculosis was on the way to becoming an older man's disease, for women it was still striking them earlier. Among all the women surveyed in the Midlands in 1945–6 there were 7.95/1,000 new active cases in the 14 to 34 age group and 1.0/1,000 for those over 35. Tuberculosis here was becoming a disease of old men and younger women. Such information could assist in control strategies.

Scotland remained a European tuberculosis black spot and was targeted accordingly. In the main cities, 80 per cent of the adult population was X-rayed in a focused few months of 1957 and 1958. In 1957, in what looked like an opening ceremony for the Olympic Games, Glasgow launched its campaign on a spectacular evening of fireworks and pipers. A group of torchbearers fanned out from the central square, one to each of the city's thirty-seven wards. Ten thousand turned out for the show that night. Five weeks later 76 per cent of the population (over 700,000 people) had been X-rayed. They were filmed by Pathé news forming orderly queues wherever the fleet of thirty-seven mobile units—drawn from all around the country, one for each ward—set up for business.

For six months before the vans arrived an 'imaginative, comprehensive and intensive publicity' campaign had been staged. Some of the 18,000 volunteers handed out leaflets in the street. Posters and banners adorned public buildings and shop fronts. 'If you have an X-RAY your name will be entered in a draw for THIS CAR', read a poster next to a shiny new Austin A35. Other prizes were a 'T.V. set, refrigerator, washing machine, bedroom suite, 1 weeks holiday for 2 in the Highlands'—the prizes, definitely an attempt to draw out the female homemaker. A letter was sent to each household and when its members did not attend, health visitors paid a follow-up call. The Glasgow campaign created a surge in the new case rate. It also

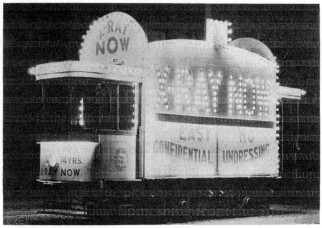

ILLUMINATED TRAM-CAR (*page* 16).

11. A special Glasgow Corporation tram, part of the city's mass X-ray campaign, 11 March–12 April 1957. With one of the highest rates of tuberculosis in Europe, the city was keen to get as many people X-rayed as possible. (*Wellcome Library, London*)

remained unexpected high in 1958, reflecting the continued surveillance of those with suspicious but inconclusive shadows, but afterwards the downward trend continued and accelerated. With a realistic therapy to offer, the reach of a good mass X-ray campaign could be a long one.

In Japan, which started from a much higher disease incidence after the Second World War, mass X-ray would continue into the 1990s, before discussion of its cost-effectiveness was seriously raised. In low-incidence settings, assessments of case-finding patterns in 1960 led epidemiologists to conclude that, important as these surveys had been, they had essentially became a victim of their own success. Where countries had a good tuberculosis service, with well-equipped and well-staffed clinics, or as in Britain, where everyone had access to a doctor under the National Health Service, they were now ineffective. General practitioner referral of those with suggestive symptoms to the local chest clinics or local general hospital was now the best way of case-finding. It was better to target equipment and personnel at two broad groups. The first was composed of those with a high incidence of cases: inmates of prisons, young offenders' units, and asylums; elderly men, especially those living in lodging houses; hospital in-patients; and contacts of children who had a positive tuberculin test. The second group were those who were particularly at risk of giving or getting the disease: school teachers and others who worked with children, bus conductors, ticket collectors, shop assistants, barmen, doctors, and dentists. The nature of at-risk groups would change over time, mirroring changes in the make-up of society. The concept of the particularly vulnerable remained even if it was not well remembered.

Self-Administration: A Real Possibility

The arrival of a cure for tuberculosis remained timely, despite the inexorable downward trend in deaths that preceded the introduction of the first three front-line drugs. Tuberculosis continued to be a formidable problem but the focus was shifting. In 1959, after several years of case detection around the globe (often using tuberculin as part of the BCG drive), WHO estimated that 'between 0.5 and 1% of the world's population are coughing up tubercle bacilli'—an estimated '12 to 25 million infectious cases' worldwide.[9] Of this total, England and Wales, at the better-off end of the economic spectrum, were still thought to be harbouring 45,000 infectious souls. India—indicative of the developing world—was estimated to have some 1.5 million transmitters. These figures, an early attempt at comprehensiveness even if many of them were still underestimates, at least aired the problem. The solution could be the use of drugs to remove the burden of disease. This would enhance socio-economic development, rather than waiting for improved access to housing, food, and education to drag countries from poverty to prosperity and out of the tuberculosis trap.

Patients wanted a cure; public health officials wanted the same, or at least an arrest of disease and clearing of bacteria from the sputum to prevent transmission. Ensuring the '100% success in the treatment of pulmonary tuberculosis' that the new drugs promised would require skill and care.[10] Work remained to be done to determine how to take the triple therapy from an experimental trial to routine prescription. Most of the early trials reported clinical improvement and arrest after three months. Continuing on to a cure was a longer job. The instinct was to give mild cases shorter periods of treatment and the 'chronics' longer. Contrary to what was expected, most relapses occurred in the milder cases treated for a shorter period of time. In ideal conditions, to guard against resistance patients were monitored for any change in their susceptibility to medication. Prescriptions could then be amended to make sure that the patient was not left with a residue of drug-resistant bacteria at the end of their treatment. Life is rarely ideal.

The initial use of one of the three front-line drugs alone (which had been the case as each was introduced) had also led to resistance in the community—among those who had never been treated but had had contact with a previously treated patient. In 1955 the MRC's tuberculosis research unit turned its attention to assessing the extent of this problem. After their survey, the next problem was to determine which drugs should be given, at what point, and for how long, over the course of treatment. The upshot was an eighteen-month treatment period, beginning with a two- to three-month three-drug phase (streptomycin, PAS, isoniazid) followed by two drugs for the remainder of the course (PAS, isoniazid). Again, ideally, full sensitivity tests would be performed on all pre-treatment sputum specimens. This involved culturing samples of bacilli on specially prepared media. How well this prescribing protocol was followed would become clear only in the fullness of time.

While the dosing rationale was being worked out it was also important to consider the best place to dish out the drugs. Initially sanatoria continued to be the destination of those diagnosed with the disease, at least for the first few months of treatment and certainly if they had bacilli in their sputum. Many would continue to undergo rest and surgery in the early days of the new drug era, although routine lung collapse dwindled. Excision, the cutting away of badly affected tissue, remained an option for drug-resistant or uncooperative patients—transients, the homeless, and alcoholics—where the disease was clinically or socially difficult to control. The aim was always to try to achieve bacteria-free sputum and so nullify the public danger these people represented. With the exception of problem patients and those whose medical condition necessitated long-term care, sanatorium stays were reduced from years to months, with follow-ups at chest clinics. It was much easier to monitor in-patients and make sure they took their pills, but it intruded into their lives and was costly. Built away from urban areas, for what at the time had been good reasons, sanatoria now became irritatingly inaccessible. Chest hospitals and chest departments in general hospitals were increasingly used to begin treatment regimes as sanatoria closed or were reused for other purposes such as rehabilitation. Dispensing oral drugs on an outpatient basis was beginning but without an understanding if this was a wise option. There was still scope to find better ways to bring drug therapy to as many of those who needed it, in the most cost-effective way.

Inspiration came not from the traditional centres of anti-tuberculosis control but the south Indian state of Madras (now Tamil Nadu). In the new spirit of global anti-tuberculosis policies, Britain's MRC teamed up with its counterpart the Indian Council for Medical Research (ICMR), WHO, and the Madras state government as part of India's National Tuberculosis Plan for 1956–61. Reasonably amicably, they would investigate if drugs could be given as effectively outside as well as within the confines of a sanatorium. Was it not possible in this country with a substantial tuberculosis problem (c.1.5 million cases), but much less in the way of in-patient facilities (23,000 beds), to consider giving the new combination drug therapy in another way, which would allow so many more to receive treatment? The shortage of tuberculosis beds, like the shortage of strepto-mycin in Britain just after the war, could be used as justification for a trial contrasting in-patient drug delivery (plus the usual sanatorium routine of bedrest, graduated work, good food, pos-sible surgery) with patients remaining at home while taking their drugs.

Just as the mass X-ray campaigns relied upon local staff to get the best out of the target population, the Madras centre and the smooth running of the trial also needed locally recruited social workers, community nurses, and health visitors as well as doc-tors. Their job would be at the sharp end—ensuring those treated at home stuck to their treatment regime. 'Carrots'—like the win-a-car competition in Glasgow—were offered here too:

small sums of money, food, and medical care in addition to the free tuberculosis treatment. By taking part in the study, participants and their families (as contacts) would also be subject to follow-ups for four years after treatment ended. There was much at stake in ensuring patients took their medicine for the full twelve months. It was crucial for their individual health of course. Should partially treated patients vanish into the slums when they felt better, but before they had finished their course of treatment, the trial would create a worse situation than the one it hoped to alleviate. Those who left the trial early would be capable of spreading drug-resistant bacilli.

The Madras Chemotherapy Centre was set up in 1956, next to the Government Tuberculosis Institute at Chetpet, deep in the congested centre of Madras city (now Chennai). Participants were chosen on criteria that revealed something of the local, and global, tuberculosis situation. One of the reasons India was a popular location for a trial of this kind was the assumed availability of tuberculosis sufferers who had not yet received any drugs. This was important because previously acquired resistance would interfere with the trial. It was becoming harder in the developed world to find such cases. For the same reason, in the USA the Navajo were singled out for involvement in tuberculosis trials at around the same time. Subsequently, when bacteriological tests were carried out at the start of treatment in India, a few patients were found to be infected with resistant organisms. They remained in the trial and provided important supplementary data. Some had lied about previous treatment to benefit from entering the trial. There had also been some community-acquired transmission of resistant organisms. These turned out to respond better to the treatment regime than those who had created their own resistant organisms by inadequate use of drugs in the past. Either way the spectre of drug resistance was never far away.

Those invited to take part in the Madras study came via diagnostic facilities at the Chetpet centre, where they would self-present, knowing they were ill, or be referred, having sought help elsewhere. In either case their disease was already in quite an advanced state—since this was typical for this population, it made sense to recruit patients this way. It was in marked contrast to the pattern among those increasingly enrolled in, say, the MRC's trials and surveys in Britain, picked up via mass radiography. The tuberculous populations of the developed as opposed to the developing world were increasingly divergent. In the later 1950s India's National Sample Survey would reveal that, while the tuberculosis problem was certainly an urban one, it was also serious in the countryside, where 80 per cent of the cases were now found to occur. Here there were extremely limited in-patient facilities, nor was it practical or financially viable to create them. Establishing a system that could work everywhere and without hospitalization was crucial to a viable national tuberculosis control programme. Although it had been tested in the city, what worked there should work for India's rural hinterlands, and similarly everywhere in the developing world. There was much to be learned from the 193 people (96 at home and 97 in the sanatorium) initially given the two drugs isoniazid and sodium PAS (the sodium salt of PAS) over the course of the trial.

While the sanatorium patients received the benefits and endured the confinement of being cared for in an institution, the home-based patients were expected to come in once a week and pick up their supply of drugs for the next seven days. Some walked several miles back and forth. If they were too frail, help was provided by delivering the medicine or by providing help with transport. Patients received weekly home visits during the first month, and then less frequently for the remaining time, although each month a sputum sample bottle was delivered and a random visit made for a urine sample to check for compliance. Both drugs were given together in a combined cachet (capsule), taken twice a day. It was literally a big pill to swallow, but the trial hoped to guard against patients taking only one drug and not the other, which was important given the resistance risks associated with single-drug therapy. Health visitors counted the supply of cachets as a further check.

The home patients stuck to their treatment schedule better than those in the sanatorium—everyone had expected it would be the other way round. Sanatorium life was more disruptive. Comments in the official publications were tinged with surprise that this could be the case given the poor, crowded living conditions of the home group, many of whom were housewives, unskilled labourers, or badly paid artisans. Moreover, despite randomization in allocating patients to one group or the other, it turned out that more of those with severer disease ended up in the home-treated group. In spite of this, there were no significant differences in cure rates. A patient could be treated just as well at home using the standard drug combination, providing they picked up and took their pills and, perhaps most crucially, someone supervised or checked that this was happening. It was vital that this supervisory role didn't fall beneath the gaze of those planning national tuberculosis control programmes.

Patients self-administering at home were no more liable to relapse in the two-year follow-up period. This was measured by a negative sputum sample becoming positive again (showing the presence of the bacilli). The sick patient remaining at home during treatment did not disadvantage their families—there was no increased transmission risk. In the majority of cases, there was no need for the sanatorium, but there was a need for a well-run service, operating out of a tuberculosis clinic, with facilities for examining sputum and culturing bacilli. The clinic must be regularly supplied with the drugs. There must be enough staff to visit and monitor compliance and progress in a sensitive manner, one that engaged the continued cooperation of the patient. Toxicity should be carefully watched for. Funds and staff to offer social assistance should also be provided. In the course of treatment there would be some patients who needed help with transport and ideally a small number of beds should be set aside. Here those requiring supplementary tuberculosis treatment or nursing, or medical treatment for other conditions could be cared for. Compliance in taking the medication was, and would remain, the hardest part but the principle of treatment, self-administered at home, had been pretty thoroughly researched and positively endorsed.

The Madras research facility—which continued with trials of different drug regimes—was joined by the National Tuberculosis Institute (NTI) in Bangalore in 1959. This Indian government institute, founded with WHO technical assistance, was charged with making the results of trials a reality as part of a national programme. No easy project. Beyond India it could serve as the blueprint for other developing countries via WHO's technical committee reports and visits. The Bangalore facility helped draw up a practice manual and train staff. The long-term goal of the national programme, to be launched in 1962, aimed to reduce the incidence of tuberculosis so that it was no longer a public health problem. This was defined in two ways. The prevalence among children under 14 was to come down from 30 per cent to less than 1 per cent, though BCG vaccination of new-borns and infants would continue. Transmission of tuberculo-sis was to be so curbed by the use of chemotherapy that each existing case would infect less than one new person each year. This would have been inconceivable even at the planning stage without the recent research on administering the drugs outside in-patient facilities.

The national programme in India was to be organized at the district level—the administrative units that comprise Indian states. It was intended that it would be fully integrated with the government of India's health services. Vertical, single-disease programmes were unpopular. Diagnosis and treatment would be provided free of cost (as were the BCG vaccinations). Chest specialists would oversee the national programme. The district centre would provide sophisticated diagnosis with X-ray and bacteriological expertise. Staff there would work with those at the rural health posts, training them to distribute drugs and to relate to their patients.

A successful pilot ran during 1961 in the district of Ananta-pur, Andhra state in the south of the country. Thereafter its suc-cess diminished for a number of revealing reasons. Local personnel who were left to take over when specialist trainers moved on to the next demonstration project felt unclear about their position in the health-care hierarchy, leading to low morale. The intended integration had not been achieved. Patients tended to go to the more familiar general health centres. It became evident that a dedicated district centre dealing only with tuberculosis was less cost-effective than training staff at general health centres, where the sick came. Money was better spent there on augmenting microscopy to check for bacilli in sputum than on expanding mobile X-ray units. Those sick with

tuberculosis who self-presented tended to stick to their treatment. Rather grimly, it turned out that active case-finding could
easily overload budgets. Self-administered treatment in the
home would in theory use the best evolving drug regimes,
although pragmatically all those involved knew that the best
could not always be afforded and the economic realities would
determine what was available.

Staff with low morale did not monitor patients well: the
defaulter rate varied from 20 to 54 per cent. The overall average
was 34 per cent.[11] Forgetfulness, the need to carry on taking
drugs even after feeling better, and the attribution of any unto-
ward symptoms were all cited as reasons in the Madras study
when adherence failed. In Bangalore, research by the sociologi-
cal unit revealed that, far from it being the victim's fault, it was
the 'slippery slope of sloppy treatment organization' that needed
to be addressed.[12] Halfdan Mahler, director-general of WHO,
called for tuberculosis programmes to respond to a 'felt-need'
by 'making effective services available to all those who already
suffer and who are prepared to accept help'.[13]

So, while India's early attempts had been mixed, countries
pressed ahead with their national programmes as research into
the best way to deliver tuberculosis chemotherapy continued.
Could it be made easier and cheaper? PAS was the more expensive of the PAS/isoniazid combination. Could it be given alone?
Further trials in Madras showed that it was much better to use
both drugs as the two had a complementary effect on each other
in the body, as well as attacking the bacilli in different ways.
Care had to be taken as some people broke isoniazid down more
quickly in their bodies than others, but this could be tested for
in trials and factored in when refining standard doses. The complexities of patients' bodies—the way they processed drugs, the

extent of their disease, differing strains of bacteria—all these were called into play in determining how best to take tuberculosis chemotherapy forward in different living conditions in various parts of the world. Cost also played a part and, where funds were sufficiently limited, WHO endorsed the use of a 'programme based on isoniazid alone'.[14] Isoniazid was also used extensively in chemoprophylaxis, when it was given to those judged to have been sufficiently exposed but not yet suffering active disease, to help sterilize the body before it became sick.

Fortifying the Front Line

Find one drug, and it's quite likely you will find another. Similar compounds can be screened and the active part—natural or synthetic—investigated. Understanding how a drug actually works—what it does to the target organism to either kill it, stop it reproducing, or help the body deal better with the onslaught— provides valuable information for creating new ones. Sometimes the search yields a drug that is useful in a completely different field and this cross-fertilization of discovery certainly fuelled the golden era of drug development. Pyrazinamide, thiacetazone, and ethambutol had problems but would in time become useful. Their utility arose partly from the fact that they could be used in conjunction with another soil antibiotic, rifampicin (or rifampin in the USA), which was named, rather dramatically, after *Rififi*, a French gangster novel and film. Refined from products of *Amcolatopsis mediterranei* and marketed in 1968, rifampicin was a new wonder drug. It was highly active and easy to take. Like all the existing anti-tuberculosis drugs, it had some side effects. Like isoniazid, it could cause liver damage; it also turned urine and tears orange—it was easy to tell if the patient was taking it. Rifampicin needed to be given in combination to avoid resistance. Crucially it could replace the intramuscular injections of streptomycin, which it largely supplanted in many drug regimes where price was not an issue. Since it was potent and well tolerated it might be possible to use it with other drugs that could be given only for a short period of time. It was an exciting time to be working in the field.

Rifampicin's arrival dovetailed into moves to shorten treatment courses and explore intermittent dosing. There was a synergy between animal models, for instance at Cornell in the USA and the Institut Pasteur in Paris, and an extended series of clinical trials. The determination of 'shorter course chemotherapies' had an 'extraordinarily important international scope' involving medical teams and patients from a diverse range of countries and tuberculosis situations in 'East and Central Africa, Hong Kong, Singapore, Transkei [southern Africa], Poland, what was then East Germany, Czechoslovakia, Algeria [among Bedouins], Finland, Argentina...the UK and France; and...the Korea spinal tuberculosis studies'.[15] Most of the trials were concerned with pulmonary tuberculosis, but the few involving extrapulmonary sites in the spine, tuberculous meningitis, and lymph nodes also yielded short-course regimes for these conditions.

Today globalization is so often used negatively to denote the problems of tuberculosis but in the late 1960s and 1970s it had a much more positive connotation. It referred to teams—clinicians, epidemiologists, bacteriologists, social scientists, social workers—with an optimistic vision of treating tuberculosis effectively, even in resource-poor countries. Beyond Europe the trials were conducted with the cooperation of the national tuberculosis services and ministries of health. This was certainly an era of less formal informed consent. Before being enrolled patients were often simply offered the choice between taking the standard therapy for twelve to eighteen months or being invited to join the trial testing for a shorter course. There was also funding from drug companies. They provided free drugs for the trials, sponsored research meetings, and paid for collaborators from the developing world to attend conferences, but apparently stayed out of the trial design.

What emerged over a number of years was a syncretic determination of the best drug combinations to use: 'not just one recommended regimen, but regimens that were widely applicable in many different circumstances'.[16] Doctors and health workers would still need to judge what worked best for individual patients given their circumstances but they now had an established range to choose from. So, for example, an 'eight-month regimen, of two months of streptomycin, isoniazid, rifampicin and pyrazinamide, followed by six months' thiacetazone and isoniazid' was developed in East Africa. The 'extra two months was shown...to really make a difference compared with...stopping at six months'.[17] This protocol had the drawback and advantage of hospital attendance when streptomycin was being given. Daily attendance for injections put some patients off, but it allowed careful monitoring during the initial treatment phase. It could be useful in establishing a relationship with a patient thought likely to abscond without finishing the course of therapy. Another popular three-drug regimen: 'rifampicin/isoniazid for six months with pyrazinamide for the first two...could be given twice or three times a week' and had the economic advantage that 'some cheaper alternatives for developing countries' were possible.[18]

Variations in daily versus less frequent doses for the continuation of treatment varied between countries. Hong Kong and Singapore had used alternate dosing days, Monday, Wednesday, and Friday or Tuesday, Thursday, and Saturday, in trials and continued with this, having set up an infrastructure that worked for them. Patients were diagnosed and assessed and then turned up to collect their pills from chest clinics by appointment for the duration of their treatment. Once a successful drug schedule was in place the underappreciated, mundane bureaucracy of running the programme was crucial. Good tuberculosis nurses or specifically trained health-care workers—different staff for different situations—were fundamental to successful completion of the treatment and the achievement of a patient's sputum negative status.

It turned out that it was also important to be flexible in place of drug delivery as well as time. Patients in Prague benefited early on from the Czech authorities' adaptability, power, or pragmatism: they were able to pick up pills at factories and other places of work. On a 'skid row'—an American euphemism for streets of social deprivation—the local health authorities had recruited a hotel manager to make sure his tuberculous guests took their pills. A single example like this in the literature could inspire others to adopt similar procedures. So long as there was a specialist cadre overseeing the organizational aspects of a tuberculosis programme, what were termed in global health-speak 'multi-purpose health personnel' could deal with the patients. Thinking beyond the chest clinic to 'general practitioners' surgeries, dispensaries, welfare clinics, hospitals, factory clinics, rural health units and special treatment stations...set up on market days in rural areas' could allow the treatment of tuberculosis to be successfully integrated into primary health care.[19]

Principles and practice often differed. The ideal was that these developments in short-course chemotherapy would feed continuously into the newly fledged national control programmes. These would expand to become truly national, in rural as well as the more familiar urban areas: the hope of the original Madras research. WHO warned that case-finding should not exceed a country's capacity to treat, as this would lead to disillusionment with the programme in which patients must be an equal partner. They also warned that any country that took on the challenge of national tuberculosis control would be in for the long haul. Tested drug therapies would take a key place alongside other aspects such as case-finding, surveillance, bacteriological diagnosis, and BCG vaccination, just as it had in the demonstration projects in India in the early 1960s. In those African countries where trials had been conducted there was said to be an eagerness to implement shorter courses of treatment. It was the best way to use the resources allocated to national control programmes for each patient and to allow more cases to be treated. Perhaps the fact that there was less of a previous tuberculosis infrastructure to dismantle and fewer stubborn doctors to re-educate helped too.

Any treatment depended on maintaining a good supply of drugs, much of which came via donor support. Many developing countries with fragile economies experienced severe financial difficulties during the world economic crisis of the 1970s. War, civil war, violence, and instability intensified in many parts of the world such as Vietnam, Cambodia, Uganda, Tanzania, Nigeria, and China. Health budgets were cut back and health infrastructures creaked even in conflict-free regions. There were shortages of drugs, sometimes because they were held up in customs. Donor funding was either cut or held steady, which, with inflation, resulted in a decline in real terms.

At the same time there were a series of checks and policy realignments in WHO, which de-emphasized the importance of tuberculosis on the world health agenda. The Alma-Ata Declaration of 1978 championed integrated primary health care over single-disease programmes endorsing and accelerating changes that were already happening on the ground. This was taken further in 1979 with the 'Health for All by the Year 2000' initiative. Allocations from national budgets that should have been freed up by greater integration of services in each country didn't find their way into tuberculosis control programmes. In the switchover the human capital necessary for a successful programme suffered: 'General health experts without proper training were unable to provide adequate supervision and training for tuberculosis control.' Surveillance, diagnosis, and treatment all suffered. Indeed while they struggled on or abandoned hope, the tuberculous populations of developing countries began to slide under the international radar, resuming the position they had occupied before the late 1940s. As Mario Raviglione, WHO tuberculosis officer put it: 'during this period [1977–88], WHO, many international agencies, most ministries of health, and academic institutions were perceived to have lost interest in tuberculosis control'.[20] The International Union against Tuberculosis was a notable exception, but elsewhere, say in WHO's regional offices, tuberculosis became one of many jobs for a busy epidemiologist. Many countries simply stopped reporting their case incidence to WHO's Tuberculosis Unit—now a very small part of the Division of Communicable Diseases in far-away Switzerland.

IX

A JOB HALF DONE

Tuberculosis, it seems, began to slip from public consciousness in the developed world. The flash bang of mass mobile X-ray campaigns had wound down. Books with titles such as *The Miracle of the Empty Beds: A History of Tuberculosis in Canada*[1] were being published. By the mid-1970s 'eradication' was talked about in a matter-of-fact way. It was a false dawn and we are still dealing with our optimistic disregard. With hindsight the period of almost controlling this disease will seem increasingly short and golden relative to the problems we face today.

Immigrants and Refugees

'As the number of cases declines and the orientation of programmes moves from control to eradication', plans of an administrative nature could be put into place to standardize notification paperwork on a countrywide basis. Brisk, neat, and tidy: things under control. In 1975 this was the optimism concluding a survey in Scotland, an area of Great Britain which had shown high rates of disease as recently as the late 1950s. In the

United States statistical analysis of the association between tuberculosis and alcoholism also led to a buoyant mood: 'to attack the pool of undetected disease, case-finding efforts should concentrate on the alcoholic population...hopefully the knowledge that tuberculosis is concentrated in a relatively easily identified population will lead to its increased early identification...and speed eradication of this disease'.[2] The nature of what tuberculosis represented was changing; no longer the mass killer, it had the appearance of a small specific problem.

Various august bodies that had raised funds, conducted research, and been instrumental in understanding and fighting tuberculosis changed their orientation. America's National Association for the Study and Prevention of Tuberculosis, founded in 1904, branched out in 1968 to become the National Tuberculosis and Respiratory Disease Association. It changed its name again to the more convenient American Lung Association in 1973. Their decorative stamps, or Christmas Seals— which had been part of America's first nationwide disease-related fund-raising event—remained a trademark of the anti-tuberculosis crusade. Stiff competition for the public's purse came from the 'March of Dimes' campaign against polio. From 1966 they both had to contend with the annual Jerry Lewis telethon in aid of muscular dystrophy. The eponymous American Trudeau Society, which had honoured the sanatorium pioneer by taking his name in 1938 (its predecessor, the American Sanatorium Society, was founded in 1905), gave him up in 1960 to become the American Thoracic Society. Trudeau, like his sanatoria, had become a bit of dry-as-dust history.

As early as 1959 the British Journal of Tuberculosis and Diseases of the Chest jubilantly dropped 'tuberculosis' from its title (the broadening 'diseases of the chest' had been added in 1943). While this might be seen as parochial, with its association with British thoracic and tuberculosis groups, it reflected wider trends. So too did the bald figures presented by the chief medical officer Sir John Charles in his cheery 'Greetings': tuberculosis deaths were down from 25,339 in 1938 to 4,784 in 1957. Concerns and interests were changing; over the same period deaths from cancer of the lung had rocketed from 4,658 to 19,119. Cancer of the oesophagus and 'acquired and congenital heart disease' were growth areas. There were still 'acute and chronic bronchial and pulmonary infections including the fungous and virus diseases'—antibiotics had done great things for the bacterial ones.[3] Emphysema, asthma, and autoimmune diseases all fell to the lot of chest physicians and surgeons. These were new and exciting areas of research and practice.

Another way of looking at tuberculosis—since it could of course affect regions of the body other than the thorax—was within the field of infectious diseases more generally. With the roll-out of childhood immunization programmes and the golden period of powerful antibiotics under way, infection and immunity were gradually reduced to Cinderella specialities. Strongholds in Britain were the schools of tropical medicine. Here the new focus on 'enabling' emphasized training of health systems personnel, improving general health services, and developing innovative maternal and child health programmes.

The MRC expanded its Tuberculosis Research Unit to include other chest diseases, running important clinical trials for lung cancer from 1958. The Tuberculosis and Chest Diseases Unit closed in 1986 with the retirement of its long-serving director Wallace Fox (1920–2010), who had led so much of the work in India. Lung cancer research was joined with other MRC oncology initiatives. Two years later the HIV Clinical Trials Centre opened—an ominous sign of things to come. This new centre incorporated many of the former staff of Fox's unit. The advent of HIV/AIDS would galvanize studies of infectious diseases in a way undreamed of by those who thought this period of human history was over in the industrialized world.

Its slipping from public consciousness did not mean that tuberculosis went away. It seemed to flourish, for instance, wherever immigrants settled. The Highfields area of Leicester in Britain's industrial Midlands suffered from bomb damage during the Second World War and a rush for the suburbs by the remaining inhabitants after the war. Its housing stock was subdivided into cheap lodging houses and low-rent multi-occupancy units, where successive waves of immigrants made their homes as best they could. This was a common pattern in British cities. In the 1950s it was the Irish escaping an economic crisis at home. They were soon joined by the first wave of Commonwealth immigrants, those from the Caribbean. Later, south Asians—many from the Punjab and Gujarat—accepted Britain's invitation to solve the labour shortage. Some 20,000 were living in Leicester by 1971. The 1970s also saw an influx of east African Asians fleeing Idi Amin's tyranny in Uganda, bringing the community to some 42,000. These were refugees rather than economic migrants. Many came as families. Some were able to bring enough with them to buy up properties here and in neighbouring wards.

Earlier, the more usual immigration pattern had been for single males to come first, find somewhere to live and a job, hence the lodging houses. They were joined by other male family members of working age and then by their wives and families. Many shared overcrowded cooking and bathing facilities before being able to move to better homes. These conditions attracted the attention of sanitary inspectors who were concerned with multi-occupancy dwellings, but didn't seem to extend to considering the potential tuberculosis risks, despite an excess of the disease in all these migrant groups. By 1975 the notification rate for the Asian population (632/100,000) in the county was 70 times higher than it was for non-Asians (8.5/100,000). In England and Wales, from 1965 to 1971, while notifications had decreased by 43 per cent among those born there, they had increased by 68 per cent among those born in the Indian subcontinent and Africa. The foreign-born made up 32 per cent of the new cases of tuberculosis.

Did immigrants bring tuberculosis with them from their high-incidence countries of origin, or did it result from the combination of poor living conditions, including low income and little education, after they arrived? How real was the threat they posed? The old difficulties in diagnosing tuberculosis—long incubation periods, exposure versus infection, primary disease versus reactivation—remained pertinent. So too did the stigma attached to the disease which, overlaid with race, was an extremely unpleasant aspect of medical thinking and the popular response. The Irish had suffered because they had left their safe rural homes and been exposed in the cities where they settled, but the much more problematic, larger group of ethnic Asians were deemed to have brought tuberculosis with them from home—WHO-inspired surveys had confirmed the extent of the local problem there. The same was said to apply to the Chinese who settled in London's Soho. Of course it mattered how people once lived here, but overcrowding in the home was only one of the problems. The same people ate, worked, and slept together; it was difficult to separate out one means of infection from another.

It would be much better to ensure that they didn't arrive with the disease. Once here, it spread within the community, and potentially to innocent victims beyond, in the workplace or on the bus home. Those who pushed for compulsory port-of-embarkation or entry screening referred to the high number of chronic cases—indicating that people came into the country with the disease. Port screening, supported by the British Medical Association, fed into anti-immigration hostility in the medical and lay press but proved unfeasible. A single X-ray machine was installed at Heathrow airport in 1965, an experiment that was discontinued.

Those resisting the importation of disease hypothesis claimed instead that the infections they saw had the hallmarks of recent exposure—people were getting sick after they arrived because of 'a combination of lower racial resistance, inadequate nutrition and poor living conditions'.[4] Data for both sides of the argument were flawed and beliefs powerfully held. The Ministry of Health opted to shift the burden of surveillance onto the local authorities where newly arrived immigrants intended to live. Medical officers of health, informed of new arrivals, were to contact them and strongly encourage their participation in the health-care system by joining a general practice. Here they could be referred for X-ray and treated, tuberculin-tested, vaccinated, and educated to avoid the pitfalls of dense living.

This was the policy pursued in Leicester. Beyond making and showing a health education film, *The Health of the Bakshi Family*, the city's response was culturally muted. The recruitment and training of staff from within the high-risk communities lay in the future. Health department staff tended to be judgemental when referring to the personal habits and abilities of immigrants. While the local chest clinic and associated services—a mass radiography unit was maintained—were successful over time in reversing the peak notification rate, tuberculosis remained a part of the social fabric. In 1998, when the rate of new cases for England and Wales was 10.9/100,000, in Leicester it was 52/100,000.[5] An outbreak in 2001 at the Crown Hills Community College received its fair share of media and medical attention. In the *Daily Telegraph* Dr Philip Monk, a consultant in communicable diseases at Leicestershire Health Authority, refused to link the outbreak with the school's large (90 per cent) Asian population: 'It would be unreasonable to reach that conclusion. It is impossible to speculate on the origin.'[6] Dr John Watson, consultant epidemiologist and head of the respiratory division at the Public Health Laboratory Service, differed in his opinion: 'The incidence...in Leicester is high...reflecting the high proportion of the local population originating in the Indian subcontinent, where tuberculosis rates are high.'[7] He interpreted this as a warning to ensure that effective services for 'diagnosis, treatment and surveillance' were established and maintained. As the investigation continued, it became clear there was a shortfall in the number of tuberculosis nurses and supplies of BCG vaccination in the Leicester system. It was also renowned for not offering preventive courses of drugs, usually isoniazid, to those at risk following exposure.

In 1976 Australia wound up its highly successful postwar prevention campaign. The incidence of tuberculosis had fallen here from 49.5/100,000 in 1949 to 9.9/100,000. A disproportionate amount of the remaining disease blighted the lives of the aboriginal population—Australia's native underclass. Despite encouraging white migration after the Second World War, they had policed the entry of anyone with tuberculosis carefully. It was ironic then that this country, which had strategically kept the tuberculous immigrant at bay during these years, should suffer a sudden influx. The 'boat people', fleeing the war zone that much of Laos, Cambodia, and Vietnam had become, changed the face of Australian immigration and began a new phase of tuberculosis concern. Midway through the American conflict in Vietnam, rates of active tuberculosis in the worst affected areas of the country were reported to be running at 20 per cent. Unsurprisingly, specific fears of importing tuberculosis were quickly voiced as Australia decided what to do with the refugees.

Typically these people had spent time in camps and were malnourished and traumatized, adding to their risk of disease and debilitation. They were greeted with intensive screening and some hostility. Although Australia eventually admitted large numbers, the spectre of a tuberculosis invasion grew. The refugees did indeed have higher rates of tuberculosis than their hosts. Subsequent studies within Australia and elsewhere indicated, however, that with proper treatment this did not translate to contamination of the receiving population. Still, attitudes hardened.

The perceived threat came nearer as Papua New Guinea struggled with high infection rates. Tuberculosis was cited among the reasons for resuming mandatory detention of migrants without visas in 1992. As Senator Newman simplistically said in a debate in the Commonwealth parliament: 'we are sitting in the middle of an area that is rife with TB, and we are taking a large number of migrants from that area'.[8] Those applying for a visa from 2002 had to be sure they were free from tuberculosis, declaring so on the application form—the only disease thus singled out—and being subject to examination. It is also the only disease specifically referred to in the instructions to clinicians, reminding them they are maintaining Australia's 'achievement as a low risk country' and that in migration law 'there are no exceptions' in the cases of tuberculosis.[9]

South East Asia was only a part of the world's refugee problem, which escalated in the 1980s and 1990s. Refugee camps were originally designed to be temporary, ideally as short-lived as possible. Repatriation or asylum for the huddled inhabitants was to be achieved as quickly and safely as possible. Increasingly camp-dwellers became victims of what the international agencies termed 'complex emergencies'. These 'combined internal conflict with large-scale displacements of people, mass famine or food shortage, and fragile or failing economic, political, and social institutions. Often…exacerbated by natural disasters.'[10] Displaced peoples living for extended periods in camps—Afghans in Pakistan, Angolans in Zambia, Cambodians and Karen in Thailand, Somalians in Kenya and Ethiopia—posed a particular tuberculosis conundrum. Because it was not one of the familiar acute crowd diseases, tuberculosis had not previously been considered as a treatable disease during emergencies. While BCG vaccination for children could be done through WHO's expanded programme of immunization, and was actively pursued in camp situations, this only protected against severe disease in infants and youngsters and did nothing to prevent transmission and sickness among older age groups.

As ever, the public health risk of uncontrolled transmission had to be considered as well as the health of individuals. Any control programme instituted in a camp setting to treat those who were infectious required enough stability to ensure compliance with, and completion of, short-course chemotherapy—six to eight months of at least two drugs to which the bacilli are susceptible. A poorly run programme could be worse than no programme at all. Fail-safe logistics and strong working relationships between in-camp aid providers and host countries' tuberculosis services would prove essential. Partially treated refugees could potentially transmit resistant bacteria within the camp, take it home if they were repatriated, or carry it on as they searched for asylum around the world.

In some Somalian camps in the mid-1980s the results of tuberculosis treatment were poor. Assessments indicated that more than half of those beginning short-course chemotherapy defaulted on the programme in the harsh circumstances. Better realization of the challenges, coupled with a redefining of emergency aid, led to new guidelines to help those involved in the international relief community. That such care could be made to work was demonstrated in camps established a few miles inside the Thai–Cambodian border to serve those fleeing from the Vietnamese invasion and the destruction wrought by the Khmer Rouge. Vast holding facilities of bamboo and grass matting at Khao-I-Dang and nearby Nong Samet were built at the request of the United Nations High Commission for Refugees (UNHCR) with the reluctant acquiescence of the Thai government.

Here health workers were able to get 75 per cent of those placed under treatment through to the end of their short-course chemotherapy during the 1980s. Another 19 per cent continued their treatment in other camps. Significantly there were almost no absconders and fewer bacteriological failures—where bacilli would reappear in the sputum after being eliminated by the drugs. Life in the camps was hardly rosy. There were many incidences of brutality and facilities were kept deliberately spartan to prevent any sense of permanence. Under the Khmer Rouge, the precept of national self-sufficiency in everything, including medicine, led to a chronic shortage of effective drugs within

Cambodia. Amid the appalling conditions of their flight some at least had gained access to tuberculosis treatment they had previously been denied.

Tuberculosis in the New Underclass

If tuberculosis maintained its presence among the displaced wherever they fled, it also continued to flourish quietly in other marginalized groups—the very poorest at the bottom end of the social scale and the homeless—in the finest cities of the developed world. Indeed, among those who eked out a living or endured a seemingly shiftless existence caused perhaps by mental or marital breakdown, alcoholism, or drug-addiction, tuberculosis would serve to bring this underclass to the notice of those who normally looked the other way.

The city of New York is famous for the Statue of Liberty in the harbour, the riches of Wall Street, the glitz of Broadway, a subway that works 24/7. The tuberculosis epidemic of the 1980s and early 1990s would bring it an unwonted infamy, which revealed much about the darker side of urban life. Some of this darkness was peculiar to the city, some to America more generally, while other aspects of it are familiar wherever deprivation in its widest sense and poor health-care delivery lurk.

In 1968 John Lindsay, mayor of New York, was looking to the future. He was still riding on the uninterrupted growth in the American economy, which since the end of the Second World War had done so much to change the lives of the majority of the American people. In conjunction with his Public Health Department, Lindsay sought a policy to clear up the city's remaining patches of tuberculosis, just as one might assess a lung X-ray and plan to neutralize the few remaining signs of disease. The incidence of tuberculosis had been falling for many years, and the nature of the new cases had changed. Most were now in older people living in residual areas of poverty. These were mostly reactivations of latent disease. It was reportedly rare for such cases to infect others before they were discovered and treated.

It would require improvements in the physical infrastructure of the city's poorest areas, and the socio-economic conditions of those living there, but the four-point programme of the Task Force on Tuberculosis could potentially eliminate even this residuum. Rather than hospitalize patients, the first recommendation was to develop a high-quality ambulatory service, which would provide treatment via outpatient clinics. In the same way as the mentally ill were to be de-institutionalized, hospital beds for tuberculosis patients would close. The new community tuberculosis programme would liaise with similar programmes for alcohol and drug abuse to ensure that these recognized at-risk groups did not slip through the net. An aggressive and comprehensive active case-finding policy was the second recommendation. The third was to strengthen and encourage participation in planning and implementation by bringing in other community organizations to develop a service patients would want to use. Tuberculosis control was not to be a lone service but fully integrated with existing healthcare facilities, medical schools, voluntary hospitals, and the like. It was an ambitious plan.

Only the first recommendation—the closure of hospital beds—was implemented. Far from costing money, it saved the city expense. This was useful because the federal and state budgets for tuberculosis had both been drastically cut, and the city as a whole was in the midst of a financial crisis. Nothing happened.

Tuberculosis continued to decline. New cases that were not reactivation cases occurred only among the foreign-born and domestic migrants, and could be explained, in the classic way, as an imported not a local problem. In 1975 and 1976 the downward trend was checked and incidence rose, but this 'blip' was overturned for the next two years. No one panicked.

In 1979 the new case incidence began to rise again and by 1983 it accelerated sharply. By 1988, despite this upward trend, the winding down of the city's Bureau of Tuberculosis Control had left it with only 140 staff and eight clinics.[11] Most of the tuberculous were also uninsured, increasing the pressure on these limited public services. The uninsured tended to seek treatment when their disease was far advanced and they felt desperate enough to endure the long waits in public accident and emergency departments, for which they could receive limited 'emergency' help under the federal Medicaid programme. They also tended to move on from one kind of provider—a charity, or public clinic, or emergency room—just as they moved from one cheap rented room to another or, if homeless, from shelter to shelter, street corner to subway. The shape of New York City's tuberculosis epidemic was thus determined in part by the incompleteness of the American health-care system, which despite costing so much, delivered so little to those with acute needs.

If complex emergencies represent disaster on a grand scale, the revivification of tuberculosis in New York City was symbolic of 'massive upheaval' of 'a social, economic and political process of de-development'.[12] Here people were not fleeing war or famine but the twin evils of fire and uninhabitable property, given up on by landlords, who no longer maintained it, rented it, or paid the property taxes, assuming that it too, like its neighbours, would go up in smoke. As the extent of the burnt-out buildings (150,000–200,000 housing units) spread during the mid-1970s, communities as well as bricks and mortar were destroyed. A massive internal migration of some 600,000 people occurred within the worst affected areas, which led to dangerous levels of overcrowding in neighbouring areas. What remained within the burnt-out streets became the home of transients, alcoholics, drug users, and prostitutes with all their associations of crime and ill health. There was an overriding tendency to blame these victims for their poor health status; it was a result of their deviant behaviour. In middle-class white districts, those unhappy with the direction their city was taking moved out to the suburbs, from where they could commute by subway into their jobs. They were replaced by growing numbers of ethnically diverse migrants who often struggled to establish a secure standard of living. Amid this fluidity, gentrification encroached on the borders between better-off and poorer neighbourhoods. Bigger but fewer housing units typified the rebuilding programme, which squeezed what was available for the less affluent.

The areas worst affected by the resurgence of tuberculosis were those familiar centres of deprivation, now areas of burnout, Central Harlem and the Lower East Side in Manhattan. It was from these epicentres that the epidemic spread: from Harlem into Upper Manhattan and the Bronx, from the Lower East Side into Lower Manhattan and over the river into Brooklyn. Infected areas in the Bronx and Brooklyn in turn passed tuberculosis to parts of Queens. A study in Harlem in 1988 presented a snapshot of tuberculosis and the nature of society: in excess of 50 per cent of those with the disease were alcoholics, the same went for intravenous drug users, 40 per cent had AIDS and less than a third could count on having a roof over their heads. In 1992 in Central Harlem, the case rate hit 222 per 100,000 people, four times the rate for the city as a whole, twenty times the rate in the country, and as high as areas of central Africa.[13] At the same time pre-school children were showing patterns of infection indicative of new cases among their parents. This was commonest in the families of African Americans and Hispanics, but rates were rising among white children too. Tuberculosis had never respected colour or class before and it did not now.

In the mid-1980s tuberculosis took on two new faces. First there was a frightening new association with the most serious infectious disease of the late 20th century: HIV/AIDS. Secondly, the spectre of drug resistance, that long-known problem, had become horribly real. Drug-resistant tuberculosis in an HIV-infected patient is about as bad as it gets. The unusual cluster of symptoms that typified AIDS left its victims open to many opportunistic infections in the chest, brain, and digestive system. A very rare form of pneumonia—*Pneumocystis carinii* pneumonia—was one of the original clinical oddities that raised the alert. As knowledge of the condition evolved it would soon become clear that the much more common tuberculosis would also prey upon those infected with HIV, frequently presenting in its most rampant fulminating form. Far from having run its final race, 'galloping consumption' was back on the track.

A person who has been infected with tuberculosis bacilli stands a 5 to 10 per cent risk of developing the disease during their lifetime. For someone who is also infected with HIV, the risk of developing the disease is 5 to 15 per cent, but not in their whole lifetime, rather for each year of their life. This is because the AIDS virus compromises certain cells—CD4+ T cells—of the immune system. These immune-system cells are essential for the processes that keep the invading bacteria walled off in the characteristic tubercle, where it cannot reproduce and cause the active disease. As the number of these T cells decline, patients become immuno-compromised, and the tuberculosis bacteria can become active. Typically an HIV-positive tuberculosis patient has a higher risk of disease spreading beyond the lungs. Co-infection with other species of mycobacteria can confound diagnosis. Often, but by no means always, because of the way the disease progresses in the lungs, their sputum fails to show the tell-tale bacteria when a sample is stained and looked at under the microscope, leading to a delay or misdiagnosis of this part of their condition. This remains a problem where diagnostic resources are stretched or inadequate or where doctors are not primed to consider the possibility of tuberculosis. Sputum-positive patients can of course transmit the disease, like any other person. By 1990, as the epidemic was almost at its peak, half of those hospitalized in New York City for tuberculosis were HIV-positive. In-patient stays were 50 per cent longer for those doubly infected. The total cost in tuberculosis-related in-patient care that year was estimated at $179 million. These were once again the younger, potentially productive members of society that tuberculosis had classically claimed for its own.

Understanding that drug resistance could occur if patients were inadequately treated with the available anti-tuberculosis drugs was not news. So much of the time and energy of the MRC's comprehensive series of trials into short-course chemotherapy had been aimed at preventing the emergence of this phenomenon. Knowledge of the correct protocols, and of the importance of supervised treatment, did not automatically translate into good practice. As Wallace Fox had written in the

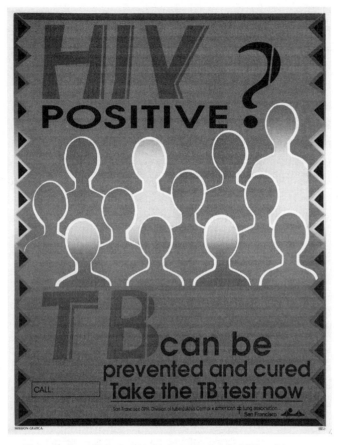

12. The new tuberculosis: an initiative to encourage the HIV-positive community, a high-risk group, to seek help by being tested for tuberculosis in the 1990s, without blaming or judging the victim. (*Wellcome Library, London*)

1960s, compliance applied to the doctors as well as the patients. Doctors had to be educated but also enabled. They had to diagnose carefully, including ordering laboratory checks for resistance; prescribe well; and ensure that their patients were able to continue to take the medication, with the support of a tuberculosis nurse, in old parlance, or a modern health worker.

Ideally this would take place as part of a programme of health care, with continuity of providers. Patients were not to be abandoned with a pile of pills for self-administration. In the case of the New York City underclass, these secondary but very important requirements were not adhered to. The financial resources, and a sufficiently equipped system, were both lacking. Beyond the rubric of the Centers for Disease Control and Prevention (CDC) and the American Thoracic Society, who were influential in some excellent but localized examples of supervised care, American tuberculosis control tended to ignore this except in institutions. It was a 'diversion of resources' and an 'imposition' to supervise treatment for all: better to spend time working out how to predict patient behaviour and medication use.[14]

At the urging of the CDC—which provided grants—small numbers of difficult patients had been enrolled in supervised treatment programmes in Miami, Los Angeles, and New York. New York had the worst completion rates. Of 305 patients identified by the Health Department as being at special risk for not completing treatment in 1984–5, only 114 had joined the programme. In 1988, while incidence of the disease continued to climb, just 93 were cared for in this way. From 1983 to 1991, drug resistance in those who had never been treated before, rose from 10 to 23 per cent of identified cases in New York City. In the first quarter of 1991, the 3 per cent of America's population that lived there contributed 61 per cent of cases of multi-drug-resistant tuberculosis in the United States. Strains of the bacillus resistant to two of the front-line drugs, isonaizid and rifampicin, were circulating and they were highly transmissible. A new acronym, MDRTB, came into use, along with longer periods of treatment and the use of more toxic drugs. Treatment was also much less successful. More patients could not be cured before they succumbed.

While the Department of Health was still catching up with the statistics, the *New York Post* ran a modern horror story, 'Tuberculosis Timebomb'. This featured the daily wanderings of a homeless, sometime shelter-dwelling, injecting drug user. He had moved from the Bronx to the Battery, begging on the subway, sleeping in Grand Central Station, and doing a bit of casual work in Chinatown unloading vegetables. All the time this man was producing tiny aerosols laden with MDRTB germs. It was one of many stories that headlined in the New York papers in the early 1990s.

It was more common to point the finger of blame at these people than at the conditions that fostered their situation in life. Equally nasty stories were written about those in prisons and hospitals spreading the disease to their fellows. They also infected prison and hospital staff and other patients, in what are known as nosocomial outbreaks. New techniques of DNA finger-printing allowed the particular strain of the bacillus involved to be traced from person to person. The deaths of innocent staff and patients were tipping points that changed the city's attitude.

A hundred years after Biggs had fought for the basic principles of notification, surveillance, and isolation, New York City swung into action and faced its tuberculosis problem at the beginning of the 1990s. There was a cultural and financial shift at many levels within, and beyond, the city. Through the CDC the federal government provided substantially more funding for tuberculosis work in the nation's hotspots: $25 million in 1991 shot up to $104 million in 1993. Along with the money came a condition. In line with the new federal policy, the Bureau of Tuberculosis Control moved to adopt a programme of directly observed therapy, or DOT. Universal supervision was in. Out went the previous personality assessment to gauge who would default, and even the highlighting of at-risk groups.

The only statistic that mattered now was the number of people who completed their course of treatment. Where this fell below 90 per cent, DOT must be used. Where programmes were more successful, the use of DOT was still encouraged to try to further improve the already good rates. Given its past record, it was clear that New York had to accept DOT to receive the money it needed from the CDC. The tension between the freedom of choice to take medication, and the danger an infectious non-compliant tuberculosis patient presented to others, swung away from the rights of the individual towards the civic good. It was a difficult shift, particularly when patients were either non-infectious or had progressed beyond the infectious stage. It was now also one that could be played out only in the most public way: 'the art of media relations in TB is the art of controlled hysteria ... You want people to be worried enough to give you more resources, but not so worried that they make you do all sorts of stupid things.'[15] In 1991 there were 137 DOT patients, two years later there were 1,282. Completion of treatment was hitting the 90 per cent target by 1994. That year the city's budget exceeded $40 million, a tenfold increase from 1988. Some of this money was used to pay for outreach workers who 'traveled to patients' homes and workplaces, as well as to street corners, bridges, subway stations, park benches, and even "crack-dens" in abandoned buildings'.[16] Pictures of these interactions made for good media copy. The money also covered an improved drug protocol involving the initial use of at least four drugs (isoniazid, rifampin, pyrazinamide, and ethambutol) designed to prevent resistance and render the patient non-infectious as quickly as possible. Better drugs were matched by improved diagnostics to test for drug susceptibility and more aggressive testing of potential patients and their contacts, in order to begin treatment as soon as possible. The improved combination of drugs and testing also increased the numbers taking preventive therapy, particularly among HIV-positive patients with their heightened risk of progressing rapidly towards disease after exposure. The ultimate threat for non-compliant patients was detention until they had finished their course of treatment. While the deterrent effect was perhaps persuasive, 'to a patient dependent on alcohol or drugs or unable to assume continuity of shelter, the importance of taking a pill or keeping a clinic appointment diminishes drastically'.[17] This draconian measure was used in about 1 per cent of cases up to the mid-1990s, as DOT was rolled out.

To increase comprehensiveness the city sought ways to ensure private practitioners were brought more closely into the fold. In 1992 the Department of Health offered free, fast, first-class laboratory testing for first- and second-line drug resistance for their patients. Free tests had been one of Biggs' incentives as he tried to get doctors to agree to notification at the end of the 19th century. Institutions sharpened up their act too. Hospitals targeted infection control. Changes were implemented for prisoners. Together with their at-risk colleagues and warders, they benefited from an extremely expensive communicable disease unit, with proper respiratory isolation via filters and negative pressure entrance chambers, at the Rikers Island Correctional Facility. Here patient-prisoners followed the DOT regime. They also received incentives to stick with the treatment when released mid-course. Homeless shelters, where some might be expected to end up, abandoned their huge rooms and provided much less crowded facilities, particularly for those with AIDS, who were likely to pick up and spread tuberculosis once infected with it, as so many were.

By 1995 those tasked with managing the epidemic were expressing cautious optimism. This was not inappropriate so far as the strictly medical terms of reference went: declining case incidence; decreasing number of drug-resistant cases; increased numbers on DOT; increased numbers completing treatment; and an increasing number of cases prevented. The expenditure on this medical solution was phenomenal. An esti-mated 20,000 extra cases of tuberculosis had occurred in the city from 1979 to 1994. If the downward trend had not been reversed in the 1970s these people would not have suffered, it was argued. The programme had also cost $400 million, $60 million of which had been spent on the alterations at Rikers Island. The price of care for those who had become infected but not yet diseased was estimated to be over a billion dollars. A good system of tuberculosis control in the USA, they concluded, was 'likely to be highly cost effective'.[18]

The expense and benefits of redressing the socio-economic conditions that perpetuate tuberculosis in communities were not part of the calculations. Importantly, the authors recog-nized that the city should think of its tuberculosis control as a long-haul, not short-hop, journey. Control for New York would involve three ever-widening circles: continued detec-tion, treatment, and preventive therapy for those in the city; improved screening and health facilitates for those joining the city from high-incidence countries; and the support of inter-national tuberculosis control programmes. Tellingly these were described as 'important, effective, and woefully under-funded'.[19] If the rise in tuberculosis, particularly drug-resistant tuberculosis, had raised the alert on a problem in the world's leading economy, what was happening elsewhere, among the poorest of the poor?

DOTS and STOP

On 23 April 1993, in London, at a meeting of tuberculosis experts, WHO proclaimed it was taking an 'extraordinary step' and declaring that the surge in tuberculosis around the world was a 'global emergency'. The USA was not the only industrial-ized country facing the new tuberculosis. In the east, Japan was facing a renewed threat after years of careful control. In western Europe, many countries would record what turned out to be their lowest ever notification rates in the 1980s. The year-on-year reassuringly downward trend was faltering in the early 1990s in the Netherlands, Switzerland, Sweden, Norway, and Denmark—all countries with very reliable surveillance and reporting systems. What is termed the 'U-shaped curve of con-cern'—decline, bottom out, rise—was being plotted before people's eyes. The upturn was often driven by one or two loca-tions in each country. Thus in the early 1990s while the UK bot-tomed out, increased rates in London and other major cities would begin to drag up the overall tally.

Everywhere the picture was naggingly familiar. Native-born cases were almost all in the older age group—reactivations of latent infections. The younger age group were often foreign-born, had a high HIV prevalence, frequently used drugs or alco-hol excessively, and endured poor living conditions. As in the USA, hospitals were inadvertently spreading the drug-resistant forms of the disease, often from one immuno-compromised patient to the next, since these were the people who most often needed hospitalization. In Russia and the former countries of the USSR, the harsh conditions of the prison system were fermenting serious drug resistance among its huge population. As the former superpower struggled to cope with the fall of the communist oligarchy, crime rose and the health system fragmented.

In the developing world an accurate assessment of the tuberculosis problem was initially difficult to ascertain. This was in itself an indication that change was needed. WHO's two-man Tuberculosis Unit in Geneva was sufficiently worried to start looking as best they could. In 1991 the unit's chief medical officer Arata Kochi published his findings: the bacillus infected one-third of the world's entire population. There were eight million new cases of disease in 1990 and nearly three million deaths, 'making this disease the largest cause of death from a single pathogen in the world'.[20] Africa had the worst case rate at 272 per 100,000. Moreover ten sub-Saharan countries had the worst concentration of HIV and tuberculosis in the world. Get in there early and treatment would be the best prevention.

The HIV–TB combination was already stretching health services—diagnostics, drug delivery, and in-patient care were compromised. It would come to take its toll on the staff too. Many were infected with drug-resistant tuberculosis by their patients, many would die, and many would spend too much time burying their friends and relatives. The greatest number of cases were in WHO's western Pacific region (excluding Japan, Australia, and New Zealand) and South East Asia, a trend that would grow ominously as HIV incidence increased here too. In total, 95 per cent of the cases and deaths occurred in the developing world.

Do nothing and an estimated 30 million people would die of tuberculosis before the new millennium. Never mind computer data woes when the calendar reached 1 January 2000: *Mycobacterium tuberculosis* was the millennium bug par excellence.

If these facts were not stark enough, the statistics on what was being done to combat the problem made for very troubling reading. It appeared that many national control programmes, formulated with WHO advice, were unravelling. Most countries could not provide accurate information on treatment successes or failures. It was thought that less than half of the cases were adequately treated, and less than half again, were being cured. BCG, which was useful for infants and young children, had finally been discredited as having any impact on adult transmission. The current vaccination option was of no use in this context.

The World Health Assembly, WHO's annual meeting, sets agendas for itself and member countries to consider and take up. Its resolutions can be a call to arms. At the 44th World Health Assembly in May 1991 WHO issued a new resolution to galvanize tuberculosis control programmes. This was aimed at current and future partners: member countries, international and bilateral agencies, and non-governmental organizations. Member countries were urged to view tuberculosis control as a renewed and urgent priority within primary care. In the face of the HIV/AIDS pandemic better-managed treatment was crucial, for tuberculosis had been identified as the most common cause of death among those with AIDS. Outside agencies were encouraged to support the WHO programme, which provided a portal to assist countries according to their needs.

The resolution also set targets. By 2000 (the original year of 'Health for All') national programmes should be detecting

70 per cent of the cases in their country and have 85 per cent of their sputum positive cases under treatment. Tuberculosis was also to be put back onto the global research agenda to overcome 'critical constraints, including biological and psychosocial aspects, for the control and elimination of this disease'.[21] What happened in 1993 was a very public version of this call to arms. The bald numbers of incidence and death rates would ricochet around the world, making front page headlines. A little of that 'controlled hysteria' had been loosed in the media. What WHO was trying to do with this declaration was reassert its role as the enabling organization for tuberculosis control—as it had at its inception—and spur on the international community. This was something it had failed to do for some time. It was able to do this because it was not just asking for support but offering a programmatic solution, what would become known as DOTS.

DOTS, or 'directly observed therapy, short-course', became the new mantra. This was what countries needed to integrate into their primary health systems—it was to be the toolkit of their national control programmes. Its attraction for donors was greatly reinforced by the World Bank's *World Development Report 1993: Investing in Health*, which declared that drugs for tuberculosis delivered by this route were 'one of the most cost-effective of all interventions'.[22] In April 2003 WHO asked for $20 million over the next two years—a budgetary increase of 60 per cent—to get DOTS up and running in the countries with the worst outlook. After that something in the region of $80 to $100 million would be needed annually to keep these programmes rolling.

DOTS was more than directly observed therapy. Its five-point plan reiterated the tried and tested technical drills: 'diagnosis through sputum-smear microscopy among symptomatic patients self-referring to health services' and the use of 'stand-ardized short-course chemotherapy provided under proper case management conditions, including direct observation and treatment'. Equally important were the three political responsi-bilities: 'government commitment to sustainable TB control', 'a functioning drug supply system', and 'a recording and report-ing system allowing assessment of treatment results'.[23] While the technical side needed to be exemplary, it was the political will that now took centre stage. Donor funds could help with hard currency needs—buying drugs and laboratory equipment, sending in skilled personnel to train local staff, and providing assistance for locals to travel overseas. Ideally budgets were planned so that infrastructure, salaries, and transport were cov-ered by governments. Forward-looking projections allowed for calculated expansion of the programme as the tuberculosis sit-uation improved.

The groundwork for the DOTS programme had been laid in the late 1970s and early 1980s in some of the world's poorest and most troubled countries. Despite relatively weak infrastruc-tures Malawi, Mozambique, Nicaragua, and Tanzania had shown that it was possible to implement and sustain tuberculo-sis control, with cure rates of over 80 per cent. There were some reversals as the HIV/AIDS epidemic and civil war hit pro-grammes in Africa, but Nicaragua remained on track. Success was achieved by joint ventures between the International Union against Tuberculosis (The Union), other external collaborators, and host governments. Each was individually tailored to meet the needs and resources of these countries, particularly the cur-rent condition of their local health services.

The key figures were the Czech, later Dutch, citizen Karel Styblo (1921–98) and Annik Rouillon. Styblo, like so many of the dedicated tuberculosis staff of his and earlier generations around the world, had suffered from the disease. It began while he was imprisoned and subject to hard labour in the Mauthausen concentration camp in Austria during the Second World War. Styblo led The Union's Tuberculosis Surveillance Research Unit from its inception in 1966. His epidemiological work in Czechoslovakia established an important framework for estimating the disease burden, which has only recently been revised on the basis of much greater knowledge. He was invited by the World Bank to take his methodology into China in 1990, where his vast pilot project in urban Bejing and rural Hebei province was sufficiently successful that the hard-nosed bank agreed to loans to support an expanded project. This covered thirteen of China's thirty-one provinces and lasted until 2001. Although it had not been the intention, Styblo and his colleagues' work now formed the blueprint for WHO's, and with it the global community's, renewed drive against tuberculosis.

WHO's call to arms in 1993 was a success, or at least the money flowed in: external funding for tuberculosis control, including aid as gifts and loans, increased from $16 million in 1990 to $50 million in 1996. In 1994 WHO launched its 'Framework for Effective TB Control', repackaged, or rather branded, a year later as DOTS. Tuberculosis might not have been on everyone's lips, but the murmur was growing. It began to be talked, written, and blogged about. Harrowing pictures of the disease's victims appeared on websites, visceral reminders of what happens to the body. DOTS has been described as 'one of the most well known brands in health'.[24] Branding smacks of commercialism rather than the detachment traditionally associated with international aid for health. Such niceties are less to the fore than they used to be. The private sector having accepted responsibility as active partners, not just philanthropists, suggested that commercial ideals could work. 'Performance-based funding', developed from corporate models, might help assess the way aid monies are spent in the face of corruption. Corruption remains a worrying drain on so much aid funding.

Image may not quite be all, but it is extremely important. Global health aid had become a highly competitive environment. In particular, tuberculosis control would have to compete with funding for HIV/AIDS projects, until the realization that mutual programmes for these two diseases were much more effective. Prevention of HIV came to be seen as a key to tuberculosis control; care of the tuberculous, and through this care prevention of its transmission, would reward those running HIV/AIDS programmes. The change from competition to cooperation would be a marked difference between the 1990s and the 2000s.

In a competitive market one must be aware of exactly what progress is being made. Time was running on the targets announced in 1991 to be realized by 2000. WHO responded by setting up its TB Surveillance and Monitoring project in 1995 to assess how well national programmes were performing. Such assessments had been among the weakest parts of past policies, and this recognition represented an important conceptual shift.

While the request for information was successful, the results of the national programmes were disappointing. Despite what seemed a foolproof brand, DOTS was not reaching those it needed to, especially in the twenty-two highest-burden countries, home to 80 per cent of the world's cases. In 1996 only about 11 per cent of cases were being treated this way; almost nine out of ten patients remained untreated or were treated by a different method. In parts of the Russian Federation, they stuck to their long-held belief in hospitalization, continued use of extensive surgery, and ad hoc drug prescriptions, 'tailored' to patients' needs, but without resistance testing. External experts, and some within the country, considered this as promoting yet more serious resistance without cure. In China, beyond the DOTS area with its free treatment, patients bought what drugs they could afford after a visit to a private practitioner. They were often expensive and of poor quality.

WHO looked at ways to strengthen the DOTS programme and increase its effectiveness. Another assessment committee in 1998 provided a further set of recommendations, including the forging of policy loops, fed by positive and negative feedback. Some were easier to put into place than others. 'Political will' remained elusive. Suggestions of a 'global charter' among the main players probably took an unexpected turn when the Global TB Programme was dismantled later in 1998 as WHO was restructured again.

From the ashes of the Global Programme arose the 'Stop TB' initiative, in which WHO was a founding partner. The word 'stop' is 'dots' inverted, hence 'Stop TB'. WHO regained its leadership role 'after a transitional, uncertain 2-year period', probably a euphemism for a few power struggles. The 'historical agencies involved in TB control' were soon joined by governments, non-governmental organizations, donors, and professional associations.[25] The number of partners quickly reached into three figures. Professional associations could help with the continued deficit in human capital, which had been highlighted at the 1998 meeting. Stop TB called once more for DOTS to reach those in need. The objectives remained the same— detection of 70 per cent of infectious cases and treatment to cure of 85 per cent of these—but this time they gave themselves until 2005 and calculated an annual spend of $1.2 billion a year. As before, all the numbers were staggering: in 2000 there were 8.2 million new cases.

The meeting that yielded the 'Amsterdam Declaration to Stop TB' was held on 24 March 2000—the first World TB day of the new millennium. This annual event, to raise the profile of tuberculosis, was instigated by The Union. It was first celebrated in 1982, in recognition of the centenary of Koch's discovery. The high-profile meeting, held in the Dutch capital, launched the Global DOTS Expansion Plan, or GDEP. The idea was to enable countries to achieve a rapid expansion of DOTS. India provided a powerful example.

Between 1998 and 2000 DOTS was taken to 25 per cent of India's one billion population, a dramatic increase from the previous 2 per cent. This was paid for with a low-interest World Bank loan. The bank had calculated that tuberculosis accounts for a quarter of all avoidable adult deaths in countries such as India. The loan would in theory be repaid by the economic contributions of those it saved. They would live productive lives as a result, contributing to, rather than taking resources out of, the system. A sense of what was involved in India and would therefore be a likely requirement elsewhere is revealed by some outline numbers. Ten thousand doctors, two thousand laboratory technicians, and a hundred thousand health workers were trained. Five hundred extra staff were taken on. Three thousand microscopes were purchased for sputum diagnosis. Drugs for 400,000-plus patients were bought. Reams of technical documents were written and printed in this polyglot country.[26] Subtitled 'The Ministerial Conference on Tuberculosis and Sustainable Development', the Amsterdam meeting's declaration made much of the social destruction wrought by tuberculosis, particularly in concert with HIV/AIDS, doubly stigmatizing its victims and wreaking havoc with socio-economic advancement.

The Global Drug Facility, or GDF, was also established after Amsterdam. Its remit was to address the need for a steady supply of good-quality affordable drugs. It worked on the supermarket model—buying cheaply in bulk, being able to dictate packaging requirements due to the amounts ordered, being big enough to manage distribution effectively. While the drug facility represented a logistical approach to strengthen the expansion of DOTS, there were more fundamental problems brewing. Just as there had been a need to understand the take-up of the DOTS programme through global surveillance, so too the need to understand the distribution and spread of drug resistance was an urgent priority.

WHO and The Union established the Global Project on Anti-Tuberculosis Drug Resistance Surveillance in 1994. It was one of the first of its kind in microbiology and may offer a model for what is a rising trend of resistance to antibiotics and antimalarials. The Global Project involved standardizing definitions of what drug resistance means, ensuring that strains of the bacillus were comparable all around the world and that the methods used in laboratories to generate the data on resistance were the same. Countries designated one or more national reference laboratories. These were linked with a series of twenty super-laboratories to check, and cross-check, the results to ensure high-quality reporting. A specialist company, using dedicated software, collated and prepared the resulting data for analysis. A fine demonstration of the power of modern communications in the computer age, but one still utterly reliant on the seemingly primitive collection of sputum samples, and their growth on culture plates.

The study's first report revealed widespread resistance to one of the four drugs isoniazid, rifampicin, ethambutol, and streptomycin. Multi-drug resistance—resistance to at least both izoniazid and rifampicin—was also common. Resistance to one or more drugs was commoner in those who had been treated before. So far the survey results reinforced what those working in the field were, unfortunately, familiar with, although the quantification was extremely useful. Where drugs such as rifampicin had only been available through government programmes because of their cost, resistance singly or in combination tended to be low. This was the case in Kenya, despite its HIV problem. Where rifampicin had recently come onto the open market, for instance in the Ivory Coast, resistance was beginning to show. What was particularly disturbing was the appearance of MDRTB 'hot spots'. The Baltic states of Latvia and Estonia, parts of Russia, China, Iran, and the Dominican Republic were named and perhaps shamed. A link was drawn between those countries with strong DOTS programmes and low resistance and those with weak DOTS and high multi-drug resistance. Subsequent reports revealed both a greater number of cases and a widening geographical spread of MDRTB. 'Do DOTS and do it better' continued to be the message from those leading and funding tuberculosis control.

Since most of those who die from tuberculosis were not yet in receipt of this basic level of care, this was where the money and energy needed to go. It left a question hanging. If DOTS was the only programme on offer what would happen to those with MDRTB? If DOTS was the only treatment available to them, they already had an incurable disease. If they lived in such resource-poor settings that DOTS was not available, they were extremely unlikely to be able to systematically access alternative help for drugs that cost more to buy and administer. Merely expanding DOTS coverage in this situation was again not a solution.

In what has been described as a 'bitter' and a 'tumultuous debate' a number of positions on the future of tuberculosis control were aired.[27] Some maintained repeated courses of DOTS medication based on isoniazid and rifampicin could still cure this form of tuberculosis. Others claimed that it was a waste of resources to fund the much higher cost of second-line drugs required to treat MDRTB. DOTS was so fundamental it could not be derailed by the exceptions. MDRTB poignantly illustrated an elementary principle in disease control: only very rarely does a one-size programme fit all. There has been a continual tension over time between grand schemes, however well intentioned and thought out, and life on the ground.

Staff at Harvard Medical School's 'Program in Infectious Disease and Social Change', notably the seemingly tireless Paul Farmer, led the charge. A medical anthropologist and doctor, Farmer is renowned for his holistic view of the social determinants of health. With colleagues he founded the not-for-profit healthcare organization Partners in Health (PIH), which aims to provide a 'preferential option for the poor in health care'.[28] Farmer's work, via the sister organizations of PIH in Haiti and Peru, provided additional trenchant evidence that the continued treatment of MDRTB with repeated courses of DOTS protocols was not only ineffective: it was dangerous and led to greater, not less, expense.

It might be neither the fault of the victims, who had failed to take their medicine, nor a failure of the national DOTS programme, as therapy had been well administered. Rather, it was a structural problem. There was insufficient flexibility in the DOTS strategy to cope with the rising transmission rates of primary multi-drug-resistant tuberculosis. Patients might be smear-negative at the end of their course of treatment but not cured, as the DOTS criteria asserted. Instead they were 'transiently suppressed'.[29] More seriously, during a fresh round of DOTS therapy they had picked up additional resistance—what Farmer and his colleagues termed the 'amplifier effect of short-course chemotherapy'. Besides the suffering and dying, these people were also spreading their mutated bacilli. Often the next victims were family members. Not only did this increase the misery and distress within a household, it could also lead to families gaining an entirely undeserved reputation for poor compliance among the local health workers. Health workers too were uncomfortable, obliged to enforce compliance with a treatment they suspected would be completely ineffective. Farmer's PIH worked with such patients, providing the expensive drugs not mandated by DOTS programmes, along with extra food and support for what were often desperate people.

Farmer is a powerful advocate. His case histories from the hot spots and high-burden countries remind us of the very human face of suffering, taking us into the lives and homes of those whom he considers the global health community is letting down. On the international tuberculosis stage, the message he shared about the costs of inaction, have helped to force a change.

A formal trial of the Farmer et al.'s mantra 'DOTS-Plus'—the term was branded in 1998—involved drug-susceptibility testing and the use of second-line drugs as needed to bring patients 'to cure'. As of 2000 Peru left the ranks of the high-burden countries, reaching its targets for case detection and treatment to cure. Here DOTS-Plus was grafted onto an already good DOTS programme. DOTS may remain the *sine qua non* of tuberculosis control but in the 21st century it could no longer be the 'sole aim to which countries should be aspiring'.[30]

EPILOGUE
'There is No Dypraxa'

I began with a novelist. I will end with a novel. In 2001 John le Carré's *The Constant Gardener* was published and in 2005 it was made into a film. The plot centres on an experimental anti-tuberculosis drug, Dypraxa. Although the active molecule on which the drug is based proved highly effective in the laboratory, in clinical trials, it turns out to have lethal side effects. Its makers and marketeers want to cover these up without discrediting the drug so great is its potential if the problems can be fixed. They do not want to compensate the families of those killed by the drug during these early, unethical 'trials'. They are poor patients in the slums of Nairobi, Kenya who have no voice until the heroine takes up their cause. After the end of the cold war the spy novels with which le Carré made his name have given way to the murky, sinister behaviour of Big Pharma, which can be every bit as devious and violent as the secret service used to be, at least in the stories. Dypraxa is being offered to patients, many of whom suffer from HIV/AIDS as well as tuberculosis and who are keen to take it because, unlike the conventional DOTS therapy, it needs to be taken for only two weeks to achieve a cure.

As le Carré says: 'there is no Dypraxa'.[1] The most poignant part of the story is a combination of plausibility and implausibility. Plausible because the need is so great—a drug which could be taken safely for a couple of weeks, like many other anti-biotics used against less serious bacterial illnesses. Implausible because, despite the considerable therapeutic breakthroughs in the 20th century, such a drug is seemingly so far from reach. And then even a drug like Dypraxa could only do so much to relieve the wider suffering of the characters. For while in principle Karel Styblo's assertion (made in 1993)—that 'unlike many other infectious diseases…tuberculosis can be controlled… under any socio-economic condition, because the infectious agent is almost exclusively in the diseased man, and simple and inexpensive means to eradicate tuberculosis are available'—is a rousing sentiment, in practice tuberculosis remains perhaps the quintessential social disease. It will always need more than a Dypraxa.

There have been considerable recent successes in tuberculosis control, including a fresh appreciation of the extent of the disease in terms of those nagging socio-economic dimensions and new funding streams. There are potential new diagnostic tools for screening, and surveillance of resistance, to help with the long, slow times of traditional culture methods. In the new millennium Stop TB has been joined on the world tuberculosis stage by a series of formidable protagonists. The Global Fund to Fight AIDS, Tuberculosis and Malaria (2002) reminds us of the original areas of interest for the nascent WHO. The President's Emergency Plan for Aids Relief (2003) provides tuberculosis funds and now acknowledges the interrelatedness of these conditions in the countries where PEPFAR tries to be effective. The Gates Foundation funds the Aeras Global TB Vaccine Foundation (2003) in its quest for a new vaccine to replace BCG.

Setbacks abound too. Since le Carré's novel, multi-drug resistance has been overtaken in severity by the emergence and spread of extremely or extensively drug-resistant tuberculosis, or XDRTB. Strains of the bacillus are now resistant to all effective drugs. WHO announced on 11 October 2011 that for the first time the number of people falling ill had declined and the number dying had fallen to the lowest in ten years. In its final issue for 2011 *The Lancet* reported that the Global Fund to Fight AIDS, Tuberculosis and Malaria had suspended its 'latest funding round because of lack of donor support'.[2] The tuberculous traditionally suffer in times of economic recession and instability. Today it is not likely to be any different.

I can feel nothing but amazing good fortune. My closest brush with omnipresent tuberculosis was a BCG vaccination at school. It was just another in the series we had from the school nurse. The only difference was that in our ignorance, my classmates and I were all disappointed that no one had a raised patch after the Heaf test, which meant, yes, we did have to have the jab. Such was the level of casual disregard.

I did not lose my mother to the disease as my brother-in-law did. His mother went on a romantic date with her husband, dancing under the stars on the roof of a club in Houston, Texas in the 1920s and 'caught a cold', so often thought to be the start of tuberculosis. In and out of sanatoria, she died on the operating table when thoracic surgery was suggested as the only hope. Louis was six years old. He was watched over very carefully as an at-risk child of a tuberculous mother. He was physically fine. So too was my friend Doreen, despite being a delicate baby, who lived with her family above a tuberculous uncle, in the flat below: 'I don't remember much, just the awful noise he made as he coughed.' This and her delicateness alerted the tuberculosis nurse to ensure she too was watched and had plenty of fresh air.

Nor did I lose my nearest and dearest. John Middleton Murry, husband of the author Katherine Mansfield, did. They had a stormy relationship even without her tuberculosis, but it didn't help. On their wedding day, Murry immediately wiped his lips after kissing the bride. She could not forgive him. The pressure of relying on erratic European mail to express their love in times of great distress added to the tensions. She spent extensive periods away from their home in London in the hope of a cure in this or that resort. She died in France in 1923 after joining an eccentric spiritualist community. Here she sought serenity, after various dubious 'cures', and died of a lung haemorrhage in his arms as they tried another rapprochement.

I was not in the same hospital ward in St Mary's Hospital, London in 1995 when Paul Mayho caught his MDRTB from another infected patient. Paul was HIV-positive. At the start of his treatment, he suffered three months' isolation and severe discomfort. He remained on medication for three years. His ward mates were not so lucky; he was the only one to survive the outbreak. Based in part on the diary he kept while being treated, *The Tuberculosis Survival Handbook* was written in 1999 to help others get through what he had been through. If you do not have the disease, reading it feels almost voyeuristic.

I do not live in the slum where the fictitious Dypraxa was trialled. These and all the other uncountable tuberculous pasts remain our potential futures.

NOTES

Prologue

1. D. J. Taylor, *Orwell: The Life* (London: Chatto & Windus, 2003), p. 417.

2. *Collected Essays, Journalism and Letters of George Orwell*, 4 vols., ed. Sonia Orwell and Ian Angus (London: Secker & Warburg, 1968), vol. 2, p. 310. (Hereafter *CE*.)

3. Ibrahim Abubakar, 'Tuberculosis and air travel: a systematic review and analysis of policy', *Lancet Infectious Diseases*, 10 (2010), 176–83.

4. Ajit Lalvani et al., 'Comparison of T-cell-based assay with tuberculin skin test for diagnosis of *Mycobacterium tuberculosis* infection in a school tuberculosis outbreak', *The Lancet*, 361 (2003), 1168–73.

5. Bernard Crick, *George Orwell: A Life* (London: Penguin, 1992), p. 176.

6. Crick, *George Orwell*, p. 176.

7. Crick, *George Orwell*, p. 326.

8. *CE*, vol. 1, p. 313.

9. Taylor, *Orwell*, p. 332.

10. Taylor, *Orwell*, p. 341.

11. Audrey Coppard and Bernard Crick (eds.), *Orwell Remembered* (London: BBC, 1984), p. 181.

12. *CE*, vol. 4, p. 126.

13. *CE*, vol. 4, pp. 329, 380.

14. *CE*, vol. 4, p. 459.

15. *CE*, vol. 4, pp. 500, 484.

16. *CE*, vol. 4, p. 506.

17. WHO Report 2011, 'Global tuberculosis control 2011', p. 3 <http://www.who.int/tb/publications/global_report/2011/gtbr11_full.pdf> accessed 16 May 2012.

Chapter 1

1. See for instance M. Christina Gutierrez et al., 'Ancient origin and gene mosaicism of the progenitor of *Mycobacterium tuberculosis*', *PLoS Pathogens*, 1/1 (2005), e5, doi: 10.1371/journal.ppat.0010005.

2. R. Brosch et al., 'A new evolutionary scenario for the *Mycobacterium tuberculosis* complex', *PNAS*, 99/6 (2002), 3684–9; A. R. Zink et al., 'Molecular history of tuberculosis from ancient mummies and skeletons', *International Journal of Osteoarchaeology*, 17 (2007), 380–91.

3. Michel Tibayrenc, 'A molecular biology approach to tuberculosis', *PNAS*, 101/14 (2004), 4721–2.

4. Vincenzo Formicola et al., 'Evidence of spinal tuberculosis at the beginning of the fourth millennium BC from the Arene Candide', *American Journal of Physical Anthropology*, 72 (1987), 1–6; Alessandro Canci et al., *International Journal of Osteoarchaeology*, 6 (1996), 497–501.

5. Marc A. Kelley and Marc S. Micozzi, 'Rib lesions in chronic pulmonary tuberculosis', *American Journal of Physical Anthropology*, 65 (1984), 381–6.

6. Bernhard T. Arriaza et al., 'Pre-Colombian tuberculosis in northern Chile: molecular and skeletal evidence', *American Journal of Physical Anthropology*, 98 (1995), 37–45.

7. Bruce M. Rothschild et al. '*Mycobacterium tuberculosis* complex DNA from an extinct bison dated 17,000 years before the present', *Clinical Infectious Diseases*, 33 (2001), 305–11.

8. I. Hershkovitz et al., 'Detection and molecular characterization of 9000-year-old *Mycobacterium tuberculosis* from a Neolithic settlement in the eastern Mediterranean', *PLoS ONE* 3/10 (2008), e3426, doi: 10.1371/journal.pone.0003426.

9. J. Kappelman et al., 'First Homo erectus from Turkey and implications for migrations into temperate Eurasia', *American Journal of Physical Anthropology*, 135 (2008), 110–16.

10. *Odyssey*, XI. 200–1; V. 396.

11. Quoted in Bruno Meinecke, 'Consumption (tuberculosis) in classical antiquity', *Annals of Medical History*, 9 (1927), 379–402, at 381.

12. Quoted in Meinecke, 'Consumption', 385.

Chapter 2

1. D. Resnick and G. Niwayama, 'Osteomyelitis, septic arthritis and soft tissue infections: organisms', in D. Resnick (ed.), *Diagnosis of Bone and Joint Disorders* (Edinburgh: W. B. Saunders, 1995), pp. 2448–558.

2. J. D. Latham and H. D. Isaacs, 'Introduction', in Isaac Judaeus, *Kitāb al-Hummayāt li-Ishāq ibn Sulaymān al-Isrā' īlī (al-Maqāla al-thālitha Fī al-sill)/On Fevers (The Third Discourse: On Consumption)* (Cambridge: published for Cambridge Middle East Centre by Pembroke Arabic Texts, 1980–1), p. xxii.

3. Isaac Judaeus, *On Consumption*, p. 31.

4. Luke Demaitre, 'Straws in the wind: Latin writings on asthma between Galen and Cardano', *Allergy and Asthma Proceedings*, 23/1 (2002), 61–93, at 63.

5. Quoted in Frank Barlow, 'The King's Evil', *English Historical Review*, 95 (1980), 3–27, at 8.

6. Quoted in Barlow, 'The King's Evil', 9.

7. Marc Bloch, *The Royal Touch: Sacred Monarchy and Scrofula in England and France*, trans. J. E. Anderson (London: Routledge & Kegan Paul, 1973), pp. 56–7.

8. Antonio Franc, *Synopsis annalium Societatis Jesu in Lusitania ab anno 1540 usque ad annum 1725* (1726), quoted in Bloch, *Royal Touch*, p. 242.

9. Both authors quoted in Bloch, *Royal Touch*, p. 69.

10. Helen D. Donoghue et al., 'Co-infection of *Mycobacterium tuberculosis* and *Mycobacterium leprae* in human archaeological samples: a possible explanation for the historical decline of leprosy', *Proceedings of the Royal Society B*, 272 (2005), 389–94.

11. Richard Morton, *Phthisiologia; or, A Treatise of Consumptions* (London: W. & J. Innys, 1720), p. 88.

12. John Evelyn, *FUMIFUNGIUM; or, The inconveniencie of the aer and smoak of London dissipated* (London: Gabriel Bedel & Thomas Collins, 1661), p. 5.

13. Morton, *Phthisiologia*, p. 81.

14. Morton, *Phthisiologia*, p. 32.

15. Morton, *Phthisiologia*, p. 33.

16. Morton, *Phthisiologia*, pp. 62–3.

17. Morton, *Phthisiologia*, p. 239.

18. Morton, *Phthisiologia*, p. 248.

19. Morton, *Phthisiologia*, p. 63.

20. Morton, *Phthisiologia*, p. 67.

21. Morton, *Phthisiologia*, p. 64.

22. Morton, *Phthisiologia*, p. 88.

23. Morton, *Phthisiologia*, p. 88.

24. *The Works of Thomas Sydenham MD*, trans. from Latin by R. G. Latham (London: Sydenham Society, 1848–50), vol. 2, p. 296.

Chapter 3

1. Giovanni Battista Morgagni, *The Seats and Causes of Diseases Investigated by Anatomy*, trans. Benjamin Alexander (Mount Kisco, NY: Futura, 1980), vol. 1, p. 647.

2. G. L. Bayle, *Researches or pulmonary phthisis*, trans. Wm. Barrow (Liverpool: Longman, 1815), p. xiii.

3. Morgagni, *Seats and Causes of Diseases*, vol. 1, p. 654.

4. Morgagni, *Seats and Causes of Diseases*, vol. 1, p. 660.

5. Both quoted in Morgagni, *Seats and Causes of Diseases*, vol. 1, p. 656.

6. *The Works of Matthew Baillie to which is prefaced an account of his life collected from authentic sources*, ed. James Wardrop, 2 vols. (London: Longman, 1825), vol. 2, p. 63.

7. *Works of Matthew Baillie*, vol. 2, pp. 100–1.

8. *Works of Matthew Baillie*, vol. 2, p. 9.

9. *Works of Matthew Baillie*, vol. 2, p. 63.

10. *Works of Matthew Baillie*, vol. 2, p. 65.

11. R. T. H. Laennec, *A Treatise of the Diseases of the Chest, in which they are described according to their Anatomical Characters, and their Diagnosis established on a new principle by means of Acoustick Instruments*, trans. John Forbes (London: T. & G. Underwood, 1821), p. 1.

12. Jacalyn Duffin, *To See with a Better Eye: A Life of R, T. H. Laennec* (Princeton: Princeton University Press, 1998).

13. Quoted in Duffin, *To See with a Better Eye*, p. 108.

14. Laennec quoted in Duffin, *To See with a Better Eye*, p. 135.

15. Laennec, *Treatise of the Diseases of the Chest*, pp. 10–11.

16. *Boerhaave's Medical Correspondence; containing the various symptoms of chronical distempers; the professor's opinion, method of cure and remedies. To which is added, Boerhaave's practice in the hospital at Leyden, with his manner of instructing his pupils in the cure of diseases* (London: John Nourse, 1745) p. 41.

17. *Boerhaave's Medical Correspondence*, p. 43.

18. *Boerhaave's Medical Correspondence*, p. 43.

19. Ebenezer Gilchrist, *The Use of Sea Voyages in Medicine: and particularly in a consumption, with observations on that disease* (London: T. Cadell, 1771), p. 12.

20. Gilchrist, *The Use of Sea Voyages*, p. 62.

21. Morgagni, *Seats and Causes of Diseases*, vol. 1, p. 666.

22. Tobias Smollett, *Travels through France and Italy* (originally published 1766; Oxford: OUP, 1981), p. 30.

23. Smollett, *Travels through France and Italy*, p. 88.

24. E. S. Turner, *Taking the Cure* (London: Michael Joseph, 1967), p. 56.

25. Tobias Smollett, *The Expedition of Humphry Clinker* (originally published 1771; London: OUP, 1960), p. 52.

26. Smollett, *The Expedition of Humphry Clinker*, p. 12.

27. Quoted in Jeremy Lewis, *Tobias Smollett* (London: Pimlico, 2004), p. 270.

28. Quoted in Mike Jay, *The Atmosphere of Heaven: The Unnatural Experiments of Dr Beddoes and his Sons of Genius* (New Haven: Yale University Press, 2009), p. 64.

29. Quoted in Jay, *Atmosphere of Heaven*, p. 150.

Chapter 4

1. Alexander Macaulay, *A Dictionary of Medicine, Designed for Popular Use*, 5th edn (Edinburgh: Adam & Charles Black, 1837), p. 144.

2. Macaulay, *Dictionary of Medicine*, p. 145.

3. John Keats to his brother George, 1819, in *The Letters of John Keats*, vol. 2, p. 102, quoted in *Oxford DNB*.

4. John Keats, 'Ode to a nightingale' (1820), st. 6.

5. Quoted in 'Keats, John', *Oxford DNB*.

6. Quoted in 'Brawne, Frances', *Oxford DNB*.

7. Keats, quoted in 'Brawne, Frances', *Oxford DNB*.

8. James Clark, *The Influence of Climate in the Prevention and Cure of Chronic Diseases, more particularly of the chest and digestive organs; comprising an account of the principal places resorted to by invalids in England, the South of Europe, etc.; a comparative estimate of their merits*

in particular diseases, and general directions for invalids while travelling and residing abroad (London: J. Murray, 1830), p. 325.

9. Macaulay, *Dictionary of Medicine*, p. 145.

10. James Clark, *Medical Notes on Climate, Diseases, Hospitals and Medical Schools in France, Italy and Switzerland; comprising an inquiry into the effects of a residence in the South of Europe in cases of pulmonary consumption. And illustrating the present state of medicine in those countries* (London: T. & G. Underwood, 1820), p. 116.

11. Clark, *Influence of Climate*, p. 357.

12. Severn to Brown, 17 Dec. 1820, in William Sharp, *The Life and Letters of Joseph Severn* (London, 1892).

13. Severn to Brown, 17 Dec. 1820, in Sharp, *Life and Letters of Joseph Severn*.

14. Clark, *Influence of Climate*, p. 326.

15. Clark, *Influence of Climate*, p. 327.

16. Clark, *Influence of Climate*, p. 329.

17. T. J. Wise and J. A. Symington (eds.), *The Brontës: Their Lives, Friendships and Correspondence*, 4 vols. (Oxford: OUP, 1932), vol. 2, p. 337.

18. Quoted in Pat Jalland, *Death in the Victorian Family* (Oxford: OUP, 1996), p. 22.

19. Murger's novel began life as a series of magazine short stories in the 1840s before the success of the play *La vie de bohème* co-written with Theodore Barrière (1849) promoted a demand for the novel *Scènes*.

20. Clark, *Influence of Climate*, p. 324.

Chapter 5

1. Laennec quoted in Barbara Rosencrantz (ed.), *From Consumption to Tuberculosis: A Documentary History* (New York: Garland, 1994), p. 148.

2. Quoted in Michael Worboys, *Spreading Germs: Disease Theories and Medical Practice in Britain, 1865–1900* (Cambridge: CUP, 2000), p. 200.

3. Benjamin Marten, *A New Theory of Consumptions: more especially of a phthisis, or consumption of the lungs... Also the possibility of healing ulcers in the lungs asserted... Likewise directions about eating... and way of living in general, proper for consumptive persons* (London: R. Knaplock, A. Bell, J. Hooke, & C. King, 1720), pp. 51–2.

4. Bridie J. Andrews, 'Tuberculosis and the assimilation of germ theory in China, 1895–1937', *Journal of the History of Medicine and Allied Sciences*, 52/1 (1997), 114–58, at 126.

5. Robert Koch, 'Die Ätiologie der Tuberkulose', *Berliner Klinische Wochenschrift*, 19(1882), 221–30.

6. Robert Koch, "Die Ätiologie der Tuberkulose', *Mittheilungen aus dem Kaiserlichen Gesundheitsamt*, 2 (1884), 1–88.

7. T. H. Green quoted in Worboys, *Spreading Germs*, p. 206.

8. *The Journal of Marie Bashkirtseff*, trans. Mathilde Blind (London: Cassell & Co., 1890), p. 573 (Tuesday, 26 Dec. 1882).

9. *Journal of Marie Bashkirtseff*, p. 629 (Saturday, 15 Sept. 1883).

10. Gillian Cronje, 'Tuberculosis and mortality decline in England and Wales, 1851–1910', in Robert Woods and John Woodward (eds.), *Urban Disease and Mortality in Nineteenth Century England* (London: Batsford Academic and Educational, 1984), p. 83.

11. Michael Worboys, 'Before McKeown: explaining the decline of tuberculosis in Britain, 1880–1930', in Flurin Condrau and Michael Worboys (eds.), *Tuberculosis Then and Now: Perspectives on the History of an Infectious Disease* (Montreal: McGill-Queen's University Press, 2010), pp. 148–70, at p. 148.

12. 'Sie erklären so in der Tat Schwindsucht und andere Lungen-krankheiten der Arbeit für eine Lebensbedingung des Kapitals.' Karl Marx and Friedrich Engels, *Werke*, vol. 23 (Berlin: Dietz, 1962), p. 506, quoted in Matthew G. Looper, 'The pathology of painting: tuberculosis as a metaphor in the art and theory of Kazimir Malevich', *Configurations*, 3/1 (1995), 27–46.

13. Quoted in R. Y. Keers, *Pulmonary Tuberculosis: A Journey Down the Centuries* (London: Baillière Tindall, 1978), p. 128.

14. Quoted in David S. Barnes, *The Making of a Social Disease: Tuberculosis in Nineteenth Century France* (Berkeley: University of California Press, 1995), p. 83.

15. Barnes, *Making of a Social Disease*, p. 87.

16. Quoted in Barnes, *Making of a Social Disease*, p. 86.

17. Quoted in C.-E. A. Winslow, *The Life of Hermann M. Biggs: M.D., D.SC., LL.D., Physician and Statesman of the Public Health* (Philadelphia: Lea & Febiger, 1929), pp. 138, 140.

18. Quoted in Daniel M. Fox, 'Social policy and city politics: tuberculosis reporting in New York, 1889–1900', *Bulletin of the History of Medicine*, 49/2 (1975), 173.

Chapter 6

1. C. W. Domville-Fife, *Things Seen in Switzerland in Winter* (London: Seeley, Service & Co., 1926), p. 106.

2. F. Rufenacht Walters, *Sanatoria for Consumptives in Various Parts of the World… A Critical and Detailed Description of the Open-Air or Hygienic Treatment of Phthisis* (London: Swan Sonnenschein & Co., 1899), p. 45.

3. *British Medical Journal* (27 July 1901), 197.

4. Quoted in Sheila M. Rothman, *Living in the Shadow of Death: Tuberculosis and the Social Experience of Illness in American History* (New York: Basic Books, 1994), p. 204.

5. F. Rufenacht Walters, *Sanatoria for the Tuberculous; including a description of many existing institutions and of sanatorium treatment in pulmonary tuberculosis* (London: George Allen, 1913), p. 44.

6. Walters, *Sanatoria for the Tuberculous*, p. 44.

7. Walters, *Sanatoria for the Tuberculous*, p. 45.

8. Walters, *Sanatoria for the Tuberculous*, p. 47.

9. Sandra Stanley Holton, "To live "through one's own powers": British medicine, tuberculosis and "invalidism" in the life of Alice Clark (1874–1934)', *Journal of Women's History*, 11 (1999), 75–96, at 86–7.

10. Holton, 'To live "through one's own powers"', 84.

11. Holton, 'To live "through one's own powers"', 86.

12. Quoted in Linda Bryder, *Below the Magic Mountain: A Social History of Tuberculosis in Twentieth-Century Britain* (Oxford: Clarendon Press, 1988), p. 54.

13. George Bernard Shaw, *The Doctor's Dilemma* (1911), I. 24.

14. Betty MacDonald, *The Plague and I* (originally published in 1948; Maidstone: Mann, 1994), p. 196.

15. MacDonald, *The Plague and I*, p. 214.

16. Astor Committee, Final Report, ii, p. 157, quoted in Bryder, *Below the Magic Mountain*, p. 68.

17. Walters, *Sanatoria for the Tuberculous*, p. 104.

18. Christoph Gradmann, 'Robert Koch and the white death: from tuberculosis to tuberculin', *Microbes and Infection*, 8 (2006), 294–30, at 299.

19. Robert Koch, 13 Nov. 1890, quoted in D. S. Burke, 'Of postulates and peccadilloes: Robert Koch and vaccine (tuberculin) therapy for tuberculosis', *Vaccine*, 11 (1993), 795–804, at 797.

20. Paul Baugarten, 1891, quoted in Christoph Gradmann, 'A harmony of illusions: clinical and experimental testing of Robert Koch's tuberculin 1890–1900', *Studies in History and Philosophy of Biological and Biomedical Sciences*, 35 (2004), 465–81, at 476.

21. *New York Times*, 25 Jan. 1913.

22. *New York Times*, 20 Mar. 1913.

23. Quoted in *New York Times*, 30 May 1913.

24. F. B. Smith, *The Retreat of Tuberculosis 1850–1950* (London: Croom Helm, 1988), p. 64.

25. MacDonald, *The Plague and I*, p. 129.

26. MacDonald, *The Plague and I*, p. 133.

27. MacDonald, *The Plague and I*, p. 134.

28. Quoted in Bryder, *Below the Magic Mountain*, p. 176.

29. L. E. Houghton, *Aids to Tuberculosis Nursing* (London: Baillllière, Tindall & Cox, 1953), p. 151.

30. Morihide Ando et al., 'The effect of pulmonary rehabilitation in patients with post-tuberculosis lung disorder', *Chest*, 123 (2003), 1988–95.

31. Allan Hurst et al., 'A critical study of pneumoperitoneum and phrenic nerve crush in pulmonary tuberculosis', *Chest*, 13 (1947), 345–55, at 351.

32. Hurst et al., 'A critical study of pneumoperitoneum', 353.

33. Bryder, *Below the Magic Mountain*, p. 178.

Chapter 7

1. Quoted in Baron H. Lerner, *Contagion and Confinement: Controlling Tuberculosis along the Skid Road* (Baltimore: Johns Hopkins University Press, 1998), p. 17.

2. John W. S. Blacklock, *Tuberculous Disease in Children: Its Pathology and Bacteriology* (London: HMSO, 1932).

3. E. A. Underwood, *A Manual of Tuberculosis* (Edinburgh: E. & S. Livingstone, 1937), p. 207.

4. Ann Shaw and Carole Reeves, *The Children of Craig-y-nos: Life in a Welsh Tuberculosis Sanatorium 1911–1959* (London: Wellcome Trust Centre at UCL, 2009), p. 136.

5. Taliaferro Clark, 'Prophylaxis against tuberculosis in childhood and infancy', *American Journal of Public Health*, 13/12 (1923), 1063.

6. Quoted in Cynthia A. Connolly, *Saving Sickly Children: The Tuberculosis Preventorium in American Life, 1909–1970* (New Brunswick, NJ: Rutgers University Press, 2008), p. 1.

7. Edward Courtenay and Frederick Hobday, *Manual of the Practice of Veterinary Medicine* (London: Baillière, Tindall & Cox, 1913), p. 449.

8. Quoted in Lynda Bryder, '"We shall not find salvation in inoculation": BCG vaccination in Scandinavia, Britain and the USA, 1921–1960', *Social Science & Medicine*, 49 (1999), 1157–67, at 1163.

9. Quoted in Bryder, '"We shall not find salvation in inoculation"', 1163.

10. *Meyer's Encyclopedia*, vol. 10 (1907), p. 28, quoted in Sander Gilman, *Franz Kafka, the Jewish Patient* (New York: Routledge, 1995), p. 242.

11. Quoted in Gilman, *Franz Kafka*, p. 212.

12. Paul Weindling, *Health, Race and German Politics between National Unification and Nazism, 1870–1945* (Cambridge: CUP, 1989), p. 548.

13. Quoted in Mark Harrison and Michael Worboys, 'A disease of civilization: tuberculosis in Britain, Africa and India, 1900–39', in L. Marks and M. Worboys (eds.), *Migrants, Minorities and Health: Historical and Contemporary Studies* (London: Routledge, 1997), pp. 93–124, at p. 105.

Chapter 8

1. William Kingston, 'Streptomycin, Schatz v. Waksman, and the balance of credit for discovery', *Journal of the History of Medicine and Allied Sciences*, 59/3 (2004), 441–62, at 444.

2. H. Boyd Woodruff, 'A soil microbiologist's odyssey', *Annual Review of Microbiology*, 35 (1981), 1–28, at 7.

3. J. B. Coates (ed.), *Internal Medicine in World War II*, vol. 2: *Infectious Diseases* (Washington, DC: Office of the Surgeon General, Department of the Army, 1963), p. 332.

4. Marc Daniels, 'Tuberculosis in Europe during and after the Second World War', *British Medical Journal* (19 Nov. 1949), 1135–40, at 1137.

5. Thuridur Arnadottir, *Tuberculosis and Public Health Policy and Principles in Tuberculosis Control* (Paris: International Union against Tuberculosis and Lung Disease, 2009), p. 33.

6. Daniels, 'Tuberculosis in Europe', 1139.

7. B. C. Thompson, 'Mass radiography: a new weapon against tuberculosis', *Postgraduate Medical Journal*, 20/222 (1944), 131–5, at 131.

8. O. E. Fisher, 'Preventive value of mass radiography surveys in the boot and shoe industry in Northamptonshire', *Tubercle*, 33/8 (1952) 232–9, at 237.

9. J. Crofton, 'Tuberculosis undefeated', *British Medical Journal*, 2/5200 (1960), 679–87, at 679.

10. J. Crofton, 'Chemotherapy of pulmonary tuberculosis', *British Medical Journal*, 1/5138 (1959), 1610–11, at 1610.

11. 'History of TB control', <http://www.tbcindia.nic.in/history.html> accessed 8 July 2012.

12. Quoted in Sunil Amrith, 'Plague of poverty: the World Health Organization tuberculosis and international development, c. 1945–1980' (M.Phil. thesis, University of Cambridge, 2002), 49.

13. Halfdan Mahler, 'The tuberculosis programme in the developing countries', *Bulletin of the International Union against Tuberculosis*, 37 (1966), 77–62, at 78.

14. Dr H. Mahler, Joint Committee on Health Policy, Thirteenth Session, Minutes of the First Meeting (Restricted), January 1962, JC13/UNICEF-WHO/Min/1, pp. 7–8, quoted in Sunil Amrith, 'Plague of poverty: the World Health Organization, tuberculosis and international development, c.1945–1980' (M.Phil. thesis, University of Cambridge, 2002), 57.

15. David Girling in D. A. Christie and E. M. Tansey (eds.), *Short-Course Chemotherapy for Tuberculosis* (London: Wellcome Trust, 2005), p. 25.

16. Janet Darbyshire in Christie and Tansey, *Short-Course Chemotherapy*, p. 26.

17. Darbyshire in Christie and Tansey, *Short-Course Chemotherapy*, p. 27.

18. Girling in Christie and Tansey, *Short-Course Chemotherapy*, p. 30.

19. Girling in Christie and Tansey, *Short-Course Chemotherapy*, p. 38.

20. M. C. Raviglione and A. Pio, 'Evolution of WHO policies for tuberculosis control, 1948–2001', *The Lancet* 359 (2002), 775–80, at 777.

Chapter 9

1. George J. Wherrett, *The Miracle of Empty Beds: A History of Tuberculosis in Canada* (Toronto: University of Toronto Press, 1977).

2. Joan Heffernan et al., *Tubercle*, 56 (1975), 253–67, at 266; A. O. Feingold, 'Association of tuberculosis with alcoholism', *Southern Medical Journal*, 69/10 (1976), 1336–7, at 1337.

3. Editorial, 'Greetings', *British Journal of Diseases of the Chest*, 53/1 (1959), 3–7, at 6, 5.

4. Leicester Health Committee, 1963, quoted in John Welshman, 'Tuberculosis and ethnicity in England and Wales, 1950–70', *Sociology of Health & Illness*, 22/6 (2000), 858–82, at 877.

5. J. Watson and Fiona Moss, 'TB in Leicester: out of control, or just one those things?', *British Medical Journal*, 322 (2001), 1133–4, at 1133.

6. 'TB tests for 5,000 pupils as outbreak reaches 24', <http://www.telegraph.co.uk/news/uknews/1315265/TB-tests-for-5000-pupils-as-outbreak-reaches-24.html> accessed 16 May 2012.

7. Watson and Moss, 'TB in Leicester', 1133.

8. Quoted in Alison Bashford, 'The Great White Plague turns alien: tuberculosis and immigration in Australia, 1901–2001', in Condrau and Worboys, *Tuberculosis Then and Now*, pp. 100–22, at p. 113.

9. Quoted in Bashford, 'The Great White Plague turns alien', p. 117.

10. 'Complex emergencies', <http://www.who.int/environmental_health_emergencies/complex_emergencies/en/> accessed 16 May 2012.

11. T. R. Frieden et al., 'Tuberculosis in New York City—turning the tide', *New England Journal of Medicine*, 333/4 (1995), 229–33, at 229.

12. Deborah Wallace and Roderick Wallace, 'The recent tuberculosis epidemic in New York City: warning from the de-developing world', in Matthew Gandy and Alimuddin Zumla (eds.), *The Return of the White Plague: Global Poverty and the 'New' Tuberculosis* (London: Verso), pp. 125–46, at p. 134.

13. Peter A. Selwyn, 'Tuberculosis and AIDS', *Journal of Law, Medicine and Ethics*, 21/3–4 (1993), 279–88, at 281.

14. Quoted in Ronald Bayer and David Wilkinson, 'Directly observed therapy for tuberculosis: history of an idea', *The Lancet*, 345 (1995), 1545–8, at 1546.

15. Richard J. Coker, *From Chaos to Coercion: Detention and the Control of Tuberculosis* (New York: St Martin's Press, 2000), p. 85.

16. Frieden et al., 'Tuberculosis in New York City', 230–1.

17. Quoted in Coker, *From Chaos to Coercion*, p. 151.

18. Frieden et al., 'Tuberculosis in New York City', 232.

19. Frieden et al., 'Tuberculosis in New York City', 233.

20. A. Kochi, 'The global tuberculosis situation and the new control strategy of the World Health Organization', *Tubercle*, 72 (1991), 1–6, at 1.

21. 'Resolution WHA. 44.8', in *Forty-Fourth World Health Assembly, Geneva, 6–16 May, 1991: Resolutions and Decisions* (Geneva: World Health Organization, 1991).

22. Quoted in M. C. Raviglione, 'The TB epidemic from 1992 to 2002', *Tuberculosis*, 83 (2003), 4–14, at 7.

23. Raviglione, 'TB epidemic from 1992 to 2002', 7.

24. Raviglione, 'TB epidemic from 1992 to 2002', 7.

25. Raviglione, 'TB epidemic from 1992 to 2002', 9.

26. 'DOTS coverage and treatment success rate soars in India', <http://www.who.int/inf-new/tuber3.htm> accessed 16 May 2012.

27. Paul Farmer and David Walton, 'The social impact of multi-drug resistant tuberculosis: Haiti and Peru', in Gandy and Zumla (eds.), *The Return of the White Plague*, pp. 163–77, at p. 164; Raviglione, 'TB epidemic from 1992 to 2002', 8.

28. Partners in Health website, <http://www.pih.org/> accessed 16 May 2012.

29. Farmer and Walton, 'Social impact of multi-drug-resistant tuberculosis', p. 165.

30. 'Tuberculosis as a major global health problem in the 21st Century: DOTS for all and beyond', <http://www.medscape.com/viewarticle/484121_3> accessed 16 May 2012.

Epilogue

1. John le Carré, *The Constant Gardener* (London: Sceptre, 2006), 'Author's Note,' p. 504.

2. 'This year in medicine', *The Lancet*, 378 (2011), 2063.

FURTHER READING

Prologue

George Orwell has been engagingly served by several biographers, despite insisting in his will that none were to appear. I enjoyed D. J. Taylor, *Orwell: The Life* (London: Chatto & Windus, 2003); Michael Sheldon, *Orwell: The Authorized Biography* (London: Heinemann, 1991); Bernard Crick, *George Orwell: A Life* (London: Penguin, 1992); Gordon Bowker, *Inside George Orwell: A Biography* (New York: Palgrave Macmillan, 2003). Some useful reminiscences were collected in Audrey Coppard and Bernard Crick (eds), *Orwell Remembered* (London: BBC, 1984). *Animal Farm* and *1984* are available as Penguin Classics. The *Collected Essays, Journalism and Letters of George Orwell*, 4 vols., ed. Sonia Orwell and Ian Angus (London: Secker & Warburg, 1968) have now been joined by Peter Davidson's recently edited *The Orwell Diaries* (2010) and *George Orwell: A Life in Letters* (2011), both published by Penguin. For more detail on the Preston Hall sanatorium see Linda Bryder's excellent *Below the Magic Mountain: A Social History of Tuberculosis in Twentieth-Century Britain* (Oxford: Clarendon Press, 1988). Orwell's medical records from there are held in the George Orwell Archive, part of UCL's Special Collections <http://www.ucl.ac.uk/library/special-coll/orwell.shtml> accessed 16 May 2012. As is always the case with historical diagnoses, there is some debate on Orwell's condition: John J. Ross, 'Tuberculosis, bronchiectasis, and infertility: what ailed George Orwell?', *Clinical Infectious Diseases*, 41/11(2005), 1599–603.

Originally published in Romanian in 1937, Max Blecher, *Scarred Hearts* (London: Old Street Publishing, 2008) is an extraordinary *roman-à-clef* of adult spinal tuberculosis, institutionalization, and love.

For a comprehensive modern understanding of clinical tuberculosis see David S. Warrell, Timothy M. Cox, and John D. Firth (eds), *The Oxford Textbook of Medicine*, 5th edn, 3 vols. (Oxford: OUP, 2010).

WHO data on tuberculosis is available on their website <http://www.who.int/tb/en/> accessed 16 May 2012.

Chapter 1

Charlotte A. Roberts and Jane E. Buikstra, *The Bioarchaeology of Tuberculosis: A Global View on a Reemerging Disease* (Gainesville: University Press of Florida, 2003) provides a fantastic survey of the physical remains of the tuberculous, which I have used for the general picture. Helen D. Donoghue et al., 'Tuberculosis: from prehistory to Robert Koch, as revealed by ancient DNA', *Lancet Infectious Diseases*, 4 (2004), 584–92 is a useful short summary. In addition the endnotes include the relevant specialist papers.

I. Hershkovitz et al., 'Detection and molecular characterization of 9000-year-old Mycobacterium tuberculosis from a Neolithic settlement in the eastern Mediterranean', *PLoS ONE* 3/10 (2008), e3426, doi: 10.1371/journal.pone.0003426 presents the evidence for this first, very early case of tuberculosis while Alicia K. Wilbur et al., 'Deficiencies and Challenges in the Study of Ancient Tuberculosis DNA', *Journal of Archaeological Science*

36/9 (2009), 1990–7 argues against the findings of Hershkovitz et al. on methodological grounds and contests whether such delicate remains should be used to find the 'oldest case'.

Bruno Meinecke, 'Consumption (tuberculosis) in classical antiquity', *Annals of Medical History*, 9 (1927), 379–402 collects together a wealth of Greek and Roman medical and literary sources, which I have relied on for this section. See also Lawrence F. Flick, *Development of our Knowledge of Tuberculosis* (Philadelphia, 1925). Mirko D. Grmek, *Diseases in the Ancient Greek World* (Baltimore: Johns Hopkins University Press, 1989) is also useful for a wider picture. On biblical tuberculosis see Virginia S. Daniel and Thomas M. Daniel, 'Old Testament biblical references to tuberculosis', *Clinical Infectious Diseases*, 29 (1999), 1557–8.

Chapter 2

Good general histories of medicine for this period include Carole Rawcliffe, *Medicine and Society in Later Medieval England* (Stroud: A. Sutton, 1995) and Nancy Siraisi, *Medieval & Early Renaissance Medicine: An Introduction to Knowledge and Practice* (Chicago: University of Chicago Press, 1990). Charlotte A. Roberts and Jane E. Buikstra, *The Bioarchaeology of Tuberculosis: A Global View on a Reemerging Disease* (Gainesville: University Press of Florida, 2003) remains a key source for the medieval period too and provides the detailed numbers of exhumed cases, etc. referred to in this chapter unless otherwise indicated.

The 9th- to 10th-century *Kitāb al-Hummayāt li-Ishāq ibn Sulaymān al-Isrā' īlī (al-Maqāla al-thālitha Fī al-sill)/On Fevers (The Third Discourse: On Consumption)* of Isaac Judaeus has been edited and translated with a fine introduction and notes by J. D. Latham and H. D. Isaacs (Cambridge: published for the Cambridge

Middle East Centre by Pembroke Arabic Texts, 1980–1). Luke Demaitre, 'Straws in the wind: Latin writings on asthma between Galen and Cardano', *Allergy and Asthma Proceedings*, 23/1 (2002), 59–93 is useful on lung problems more generally. On medieval China see Liu Ts'un-Yan, 'The Taoists' knowledge of tuberculosis in the twelfth century', *T'oung Pao*, 2nd ser., 57/5 (1971), 285–301.

Scrofula is the subject of the wonderful Marc Bloch, *The Royal Touch: Sacred Monarchy and Scrofula in England and France*, trans. J. E. Anderson (London: Routledge & Kegan Paul, 1973), although Frank Barlow, 'The King's Evil', *English Historical Review*, 95 (1980), 3–27 provides some amendments to Bloch's chronology. For the great use of snails as a cure for scrofula see Kenelm Digby, *Choice and Experimented Receipts in Physick and Chirurgery* (London: Henry Brome, 1675), p. 53.

For the Italian death registers see Ann G. Carmichael, 'The health status of Florentines in the fifteenth century', in Marcel Tetel et al. (eds.), *Life and Death in Fifteenth Century Florence* (Durham, NC: Duke University Press, 1989), pp. 28–45. For the French see Laurence Brockliss and Colin Jones, *The Medical World of Early Modern France* (Oxford: Clarendon Press, 1997). On the idea of a consumptive death as a good death see Clark Lawlor, *Consumption and Literature: The Making of the Romantic Disease* (Basingstoke: Palgrave Macmillan, 2006), which explains beautifully how and why this notion arose from the early modern period, and why it was a fallacy.

Richard Morton's monumental *Phthisiologia; or, A Treatise of Consumptions. Wherein the difference, nature, causes, signs, and cure of all sorts of consumptions are explained. Containing three books: I. Of the original consumptions from the whole habit of the body. II. Of an original consumption of the lungs. III. Of symptomatical consumptions, or such as are the effects of some other distempers. Illustrated by particular cases, and observations added to every book. With a compleat table of the most remarkable things*, translated from the Latin original of 1689 (2nd, corrected edn, London: W. & J. Innys, 1720). See also R. Y. Keers, 'Richard Morton (1837–98) and his phthisiologia', *Thorax*, 37 (1982), 26–31; R. R. Trial, 'Richard Morton (1637–98)', *Medical History*, 14 (1970), 166–74.

Chapter 3

Giovanni Battista Morgagni, *The Seats and Causes of Diseases Investigated by Anatomy*, trans. Benjamin Alexander (Mount Kisco, NY: Futura, 1980) is a three-volume facsimile of the 18th-century translation of this magnificent text. Matthew Baillie's *The Morbid Anatomy of Some of the Most Important Parts of the Human Body* of 1793 is available as part of *The Works of Matthew Baillie to which is prefaced an account of his life collected from authentic sources*, edited by James Wardrop, 2 vols. (London: Longman, 1825).

A Treatise of the Diseases of the Chest, in which they are described according to their Anatomical Characters, and their Diagnosis established on a new principle by means of Acoustick Instruments is John Forbes' 1821 translation of Laennec's masterpiece (London: T. & G. Underwood, 1821); a facsimile of this edition was reproduced by Hafer Publishing, New York in 1962. Jacalyn Duffin, *To See with a Better Eye: A Life of R. T. H. Laennec* (Princeton: Princeton University Press, 1998) takes the reader into the heart of Laennec's world of stethoscopes and diseased lungs.

Boerhaave's Medical Correspondence; containing the various symptoms of chronical distempers; the professor's opinion, method of cure and remedies. To which is added, Boerhaave's practice in the hospital at Leyden, with his manner of instructing his pupils in the cure of diseases

(London: John Nourse, 1745) is a translation of the Boerhaave letters. For their context see Lester S. King, *The Medical World of the Eighteenth Century* (Chicago: University of Chicago Press, 1958).

On travelling for health see E. S. Turner, *Taking the Cure* (London: Michael Joseph, 1967). On travelling generally, Christopher Hibbert, *The Grand Tour* (London: Weidenfeld & Nicolson, 1969) remains the place to begin. Brian Dolan, *Ladies of the Grand Tour* (London: HarperCollins, 2001) adds some nice feminine details. Tobias Smollett's books that educated and entertained me were: *Travels through France and Italy* (originally published 1766; edition used here, Oxford: OUP, 1981) and *The Expedition of Humphry Clinker* (originally published 1771, the year of his death; the edition used here, London: OUP, 1960). Jeremy Lewis, *Tobias Smollett* (London: Pimlico, 2004) is a nice biography of the old curmudgeon. Smollett was also the author of *An Essay on the External Use of Water* (1752), which set out his views on the curative properties of cold water and suggestions to improve the bathing conditions and decorum at Bath. Benjamin Pugh, *Observations of the Climate of Naples, Rome, Nice etc.* (London: G. Robinson, 1784) provided more medical details on the familiar destinations. Ebenezer Gilchrist, *The Use of Sea Voyages in Medicine: and particularly in a consumption, with observations on that disease* (London T. Cadell, 1771) describes the virtues of sea travel with case histories.

On Thomas Beddoes see Roy Porter, *Thomas Beddoes and the Sick Trade in Late-Enlightenment England* (London: Routledge, 1992) and Mike Jay, *The Atmosphere of Heaven: The Unnatural Experiments of Dr Beddoes and his Sons of Genius* (New Haven: Yale University Press, 2009), a great new biography. Roy Porter, 'Consumption: disease of the consumer society?', in John Brewer and Roy Porter (eds.), *Consumption and the World of Goods* (London: Routledge, 1994), pp. 58–81 superbly locates the disease in the society of excess at the end of the 18th century.

Chapter 4

Among the primary sources I relied upon for this chapter are Alexander Macaulay's *A Dictionary of Medicine, Designed for Popular Use*, 5th edn (Edinburgh: Adam & Charles Black, 1837); James Clark's *Medical Notes on Climate, Diseases, Hospitals and Medical Schools in France, Italy and Switzerland; comprising an inquiry into the effects of a residence in the South of Europe in cases of pulmonary consumption. And illustrating the present state of medicine in those countries* (London: T. & G. Underwood, 1820) and *The Influence of Climate in the Prevention and Cure of Chronic Diseases, more particularly of the chest and digestive organs; comprising an account of the principal places resorted to by invalids in England, the South of Europe, etc.; a comparative estimate of their merits in particular diseases, and general directions for invalids while travelling and residing abroad* (London: J. Murray, 1830).

The subjective experience of disease has received increasing attention since Susan Sontag's provocative *Illness as Metaphor* (New York: Vintage Books, 1979). In this vein I found Clark Lawler and Akihito Suzuki's 'The disease of the self: representing consumption, 1700–1830', *Bulletin of the History of Medicine*, 74 (2000), 458–94 and Clark Lawlor's *Consumption and Literature: The Making of the Romantic Disease* (Basingstoke: Palgrave Macmillan, 2006) the place to begin. Thomas Dormandy's *The White Death: A History of Tuberculosis* (London: Hambledon Press, 1999) is particularly good on potted patient histories.

Kelvin Everest's *Oxford DNB* article on John Keats was extremely useful, <http://www.oxforddnb.com/view/article/

15229> accessed 16 May 2012; see also Andrew Bennett on Frances (Fanny) Brawne <http://www.oxforddnb.com/view/article/47474> accessed 16 March 2012, and David Kaloustian on Joseph Severn <http://www.oxforddnb.com/view/article/25132> accessed 16 May 2012. Andrew Motion's biography *Keats* (London: Faber & Faber, 1997) is another place to start for John and Fanny and for the Keats circle, as well as the poetry. William Sharp, *The Life and Letters of Joseph Severn* (London, 1892) includes Severn's letters home from Rome from which the quotations are taken.

Sally Palmer, ' "I prefer walking": Jane Austen and "the pleasantest part of the day" ', *Persusasions: The Jane Austen Journal*, 23 (2001), 154–65. On the history of hysteria see Andrew Scull, *Hysteria: The Disturbing History* (Oxford: OUP, 2011), and on invalidism see Maria H. Frawley, *Invalidism and Identity in Nineteenth-Century Britain* (Chicago: University of Chicago Press, 2004).

Winifred Gérin's biographies of the Brontës became addictive: *Anne Brontë* (1959), *Branwell Brontë* (1961), *Charlotte Brontë: The Evolution of Genius* (1967), *Emily Brontë* (1971). T. J. Wise and J. A. Symington (eds.), *The Brontës: Their Lives, Friendships and Correspondence*, 4 vols. (Oxford: OUP, 1932). For Thérèse Martin and the heroines of Murger and Dumas, see David S. Barnes, *The Making of a Social Disease: Tuberculosis in Nineteenth Century France* (Berkeley: University of California Press, 1995). Pat Jalland, *Death in the Victorian Family* (Oxford: OUP, 1996) includes several harrowing tuberculosis deaths including that of Caroline Leakey. Arthur Groos, ' "TB sheets": love and disease in *La traviata*', *Cambridge Opera Journal*, 7/3 (1995), 233–60 is a fine description of what he terms one of the great 'coughers' of 19th-century opera.

Chapter 5

Barbara Rosencrantz (ed.), *From Consumption to Tuberculosis: A Documentary History* (New York: Garland, 1994) is an excellent collection of reprints of primary sources for the 19th and 20th centuries in this crucial period as the disease is remade.

On germs, germ theory, and Robert Koch see the excellent studies by Michael Worboys, *Spreading Germs: Disease Theories and Medical Practice in Britain, 1865–1900* (Cambridge: CUP, 2000) and Christoph Gradmann, *Laboratory Disease: Robert Koch's Medical Bacteriology*, trans. Elborg Forster (Baltimore: Johns Hopkins University Press, 2009). On tuberculosis germs in the home see Nancy Tomes, *The Gospel of Germs: Men, Women, and the Microbe in American Life* (Cambridge, MA: Harvard University Press, 1998). For translations of Robert Koch's tuberculosis papers see *Essays of Robert Koch*, trans. K. Codell Carter (New York: Greenwood, 1987).

Benjamin Marten described his ideas in *A New Theory of Consumptions: more especially of a phthisis, or consumption of the lungs...Also the possibility of healing ulcers in the lungs asserted... Likewise directions about eating...and way of living in general, proper for consumptive persons* (London: R. Knaplock, A. Bell, J. Hooke, & C. King, 1720), where he also describes the standard treatments of the time. Bridie J. Andrews, 'Tuberculosis and the assimilation of germ theory in China, 1895–1937', *Journal of the History of Medicine and Allied Sciences*, 52/1(1997), 114–58 describes the arrival of germ theory in China.

The Journal of Marie Bashkirtseff, trans. Mathilde Blind (London: Cassell & Co., 1890) contains many poignant entries charting her worsening health with visits to doctors and the attempts to improve her condition. See David S. Barnes, *The Making of a*

Social Disease: Tuberculosis in Nineteenth Century France (Berkeley: University of California Press, 1995) for the French responses and also Allan Mitchell, 'An inexact science: the statistics of tuberculosis in late nineteenth-century France', *Social History of Medicine*, 3/3 (1990): 387–403.

Gillian Cronje, 'Tuberculosis and mortality decline in England and Wales, 1851–1910', in Robert Woods and John Woodward (eds.), *Urban Disease and Mortality in Nineteenth Century England* (London: Batsford Academic and Educational, 1984), pp. 79–101 provides statistics, as does Michael Worboys, 'Before McKeown: explaining the decline of tuberculosis in Britain, 1880–1930', in Flurin Condrau and Michael Worboys (eds.), *Tuberculosis Then and Now: Perspectives on the History of an Infectious Disease* (Montreal: McGill-Queen's University Press, 2010), pp. 148–70. Details of the tuberculosis epidemic around the world are found in numerous papers and monographs including Veran Blinn Reber, 'Blood, coughs, and fever: tuberculosis and the working class of Buenos Aires, Argentina', *Social History of Medicine*, 12/1 (1999), 73–100 (Reber discussed the hard working conditions in the bakeries); Diego Armus, *The Ailing City: Health, Tuberculosis, and Culture in Buenos Aires, 1870–1950* (Durham, NC: Duke University Press, 2011); William Johnston, *The Modern Epidemic: A History of Tuberculosis in Japan* (Cambridge, MA: Council on East Asian Studies, Harvard University, 1995) and 'A genealogy of tubercular diseases in Japan', *Social History of Medicine*, 7/2 (1994), 247–67; K. David Patterson, 'Mortality in late tsarist Russia: a reconnaissance', *Social History of Medicine*, 8/2 (1995), 179–210; Jörg Vögele, *Urban Mortality Change in England and Germany, 1870–1913* (Liverpool: Liverpool University Press, 1998). Others are listed elsewhere as appropriate.

Robert Philip's *Collected Papers on Tuberculosis* (London: OUP, 1937) charts his career as a tuberculosis expert. On Biggs see C.-E. A. Winslow, *The Life of Hermann M. Biggs: M.D., D.SC., LL.D., Physician and Statesman of the Public Health* (Philadelphia: Lea & Febiger, 1929) and Daniel M. Fox, 'Social policy and city politics: tuberculosis reporting in New York, 1889–1900', *Bulletin of the History of Medicine*, 49/2 (1975), 169–195. The work of both (and much more) is discussed in R. Y. Keers, *Pulmonary Tuberculosis: A Journey Down the Centuries* (London: Baillière Tindall, 1978) and F. B. Smith, *The Retreat of Tuberculosis 1850–1950* (London: Croom Helm, 1988).

Chapter 6

Thomas Mann, *Magic Mountain* remains the classic novel of the elite tuberculosis sanatorium and certain values in Europe before the watershed of the First World War. A. E. Eillis, *The Rack* (London: Heinemann, 1958; reissued by Penguin, 1979) tells of life after the Second World War.

Mann's novel inspired the title of Linda Bryder, *Below the Magic Mountain: A Social History of Tuberculosis in Twentieth-Century Britain* (Oxford: Clarendon Press, 1988), a wonderfully rich look at the provisions and nature of the care within and without the institution in the first half of the 20th century. F. B. Smith, *The Retreat of Tuberculosis 1850–1950* (London: Croom Helm, 1988) covers some of the same material. A. Adams, K. Schwartzman, and D. Theodore, 'Collapse and Expand: architecture and tuberculosis therapy in Montreal, 1909, 1922, 1954', *Technology and Culture*, 49/4 (2008), 908–42 provides a detailed description of changing sanatorium design and the care offered there. Among the excellent histories of sanatorium life and its lived experience in North

America see Sheila M. Rothman, *Living in the Shadow of Death: Tuberculosis and the Social Experience of Illness in American History* (New York: Basic Books, 1994); Barbara Bates, *Bargaining for Life: A Social History of Tuberculosis, 1876–1938* (Philadelphia: University of Philadelphia Press, 1992); Katherine McCuaig, *The Weariness, the Fever, and the Fret: The Campaign against Tuberculosis in Canada, 1900–1950* (Montreal: McGill-Queen's University Press, 1999); and Katherine Ott, *Fevered Lives: Tuberculosis in American Culture since 1870* (Cambridge, MA: Harvard University Press, 1996).

Betty MacDonald, *The Plague and I* (originally published in 1948; Maidstone: Mann, 1994) brings the personal side of sanatorium life and the surgical tuberculosis treatment to the fore. I found Frank McLynn, *Robert Louis Stevenson* (London: Pimlico, 1994) a useful biography. For other patient experiences featured here see Sandra Stanley Holton, 'To live "through one's own powers": British medicine, tuberculosis and "invalidism" in the life of Alice Clark (1874–1934)', *Journal of Women's History*, 11 (1999), 75–96.

F. Rufenacht Walters, *Sanatoria for Consumptives in Various Parts of the World... A Critical and Detailed Description of The Open-Air or Hygienic Treatment of Phthisis* (London: Swan Sonnenschein & Co., 1899) ran through two further editions in 1901 and 1905 before becoming *Sanatoria for the Tuberculous; including a description of many existing institutions and of sanatorium treatment in pulmonary tuberculosis* (London: George Allen, 1913). Edward L. Trudeau wrote *An Autobiography* (Philadelphia: Lea & Febiger, 1916). See also David L. Ellison, *Healing Tuberculosis in the Woods: Medicine and Science at the end of the Nineteenth Century* (Westport, CT: Greenwood, 1994).

Christoph Gradmann explores Koch's tuberculin in 'A harmony of illusions: clinical and experimental testing of Robert

Koch's tuberculin 1890–1900', *Studies in History and Philosophy of Biological and Biomedical Sciences*, 35 (2004), 465–81 and 'Robert Koch and the white death: from tuberculosis to tuberculin', *Microbes and Infection*, 8 (2006), 294–301. See also D. S. Burke, 'Of postulates and peccadilloes: Robert Koch and vaccine (tuberculin) therapy for tuberculosis', *Vaccine*, 11 (1993), 795–804; Cristina Vilaplana and Pere-Joan Cardona, 'Tuberculin immunotherapy: its history and lessons to be learned', *Microbes and Infection*, 12 (2010), 99–105.

E. A. Underwood, *A Manual of Tuberculosis* (Edinburgh: E. & S. Livingstone, 1937) and L. E. Houghton, *Aids to Tuberculosis Nursing* (London: Bailllière, Tindall & Cox, 1953) provide useful details on contemporary care of the tuberculous.

Chapter 7

Cynthia A. Connolly, *Saving Sickly Children; The Tuberculosis Preventorium in American Life, 1909–1970* (New Brunswick, NJ: Rutgers University Press, 2008) describes the development of these institutions. For a first-hand account of life there see Eileen Simpson, *Orphans Real and Imaginary* (New York: Weidenfeld & Nicolson, 1987). Listen to Mike Emanuel as he discusses the history of the Open Air School Movement <http://ah.brookes. ac.uk/historyofmedicine/podcast/the_open_air_school_ movement_in_the_first_half_of_the_twentieth_century/ accessed 16 May 2012. In the English context the oral history by Ann Shaw and Carole Reeves, *The Children of Craig-y-nos: Life in a Welsh Tuberculosis Sanatorium 1911–1959* (London: Wellcome Trust Centre at UCL, 2009) is evocative; it is available online at <http:// www.ucl.ac.uk/histmed/downloads/the_children_of_craig_y_ nos.pdf> accessed 16 May 2012. John W. S. Blacklock, *Tuberculous*

Disease in Children: Its Pathology and Bacteriology (London: HMSO, 1932) provided a useful review of contemporary research.

Keir Waddington, *The Bovine Scourge: Meat, Tuberculosis and Public Health, 1850–1914* (Woodbridge: Boydell Press, 2006); and also his 'To stamp out "so terrible a malady": bovine tuberculosis and tuberculin testing in Britain, 1890–1939', *Medical History*, 48 (2004), 29–48; Peter J. Atkins, 'White poison? The social consequences of milk consumption, 1850–1930', *Social History of Medicine*, 5/2 (1992), 207–27; and Barbara Rosenkrantz, 'The trouble with bovine tuberculosis', *Bulletin of the History of Medicine*, 59/2 (1985), 155–75 cover important aspects of the milk, meat, and tuberculosis problem.

Lynda Bryder, '"We shall not find salvation in inoculation": BCG vaccination in Scandinavia, Britain and the USA, 1921–1960', *Social Science & Medicine*, 49 (1999), 1157–67 is a fine review of who does and does not takes up BCG and why.

Paul Weindling, *Health, Race and German Politics between National Unification and Nazism, 1870–1945* (Cambridge: CUP, 1989) describes the fate of the tuberculous as the Nazis come to power. Sander Gilman, *Franz Kafka, the Jewish Patient* (New York: Routledge, 1995) is an excellent place to begin to understand this man and his ill health.

On tuberculosis and race in the USA see Marion M. Tochia, 'Tuberculosis among American Negroes: medical research on a racial disease, 1830–1950', *Journal of the History of Medicine and Allied Sciences*, 20/3 (1977), 253–79, and Georgina D. Feldberg, *Disease and Class: Tuberculosis and the Shaping of Modern North American Society* (New Brunswick, NJ: Rutgers University Press, 1995). Randall Packard's *White Plague, Black Labor: Tuberculosis and the Political Economy of Health and Disease in South Africa* (Pietermaritzburg: University of Natal Press, 1990) remains the seminal study. Mark

Harrison and Michael Worboys, 'A disease of civilization: tuberculosis in Britain, Africa and India, 1900–39', in L. Marks and M. Worboys (eds.), *Migrants, Minorities and Health: Historical and Contemporary Studies* (London: Routledge, 1997), pp. 93–124 and Michael Worboys, 'Tuberculosis and race in Britain and its empire, 1900–50', in Waltraud Ernst and Bernard Harris (eds.), *Race, Science and Medicine, 1700–1960* (London: Routledge, 1999), pp. 144–66 dissects the role of Lyle Cummins and his ideas.

Chapter 8

William Kingston, 'Streptomycin, Schatz v. Waksman, and the balance of credit for discovery', *Journal of the History of Medicine and Allied Sciences*, 59/3 (2004), 441–62 and Milton Wainwright, 'A response to William Kingston, "Streptomycin, *Schatz versus Waksman*, and the balance of credit for discovery", *Journal of the History of Medicine and Allied Sciences*, 60/2 (2005), 218–20 argue the claims of Albert Schatz. For a short standard account see Alex Sakula, 'Selman Waksman (1888–1973), discoverer of streptomycin: a centenary review', *British Journal of Diseases of the Chest*, 82 (1988), 23–31 and in more detail J. H. Comroe, 'Pay dirt: the story of streptomycin', *American Review of Respiratory Disease*, 117 (1978), 773–81, 957–68.

Early papers of Waksman's include Selman A. Waksman and H. Boyd Woodruff, 'The soil as a source of microorganims antagonistic to disease-producing bacteria', *Journal of Bacteriology*, 40/4 (1940), 581–600 and 'Selective antibiotic actions of various substances of microbial origin', *Journal of Bacteriology*, 44/3 (1942), 373–84. See also summaries by Waksman, 'What is an antibiotic or an antibiotic substance?', *Mycologia*, 39/5 (1947), 565–9 and 'Streptomycin: isolation, properties, and utilisation', *Journal of the History of Medicine and Allied Sciences*, 6 (1951), 318–47.

For Waksman as historian on his work see *My Life with the Microbes* (London: Scientific Book Club, 1958) and *The Conquest of Tuberculosis* (Berkeley: University of California Press, 1964).

H. Boyd Woodruff, 'A soil microbiologist's odyssey', *Annual Review of Microbiology*, 35 (1981), 1–28 gives his own voice. This is probably a good place to mention René Dubos and Jean Dubos, *The White Plague: Tuberculosis, Man and Society* (London: Gollancz, 1953), a classic history of tuberculosis written by Dubos and his second wife (he had lost his first wife to tuberculosis).

David Greenwood, *Antimicrobial Drugs: Chronicle of a Twentieth-Century Medical Triumph* (Oxford: OUP, 2008) is good on the history of all the anti-tuberculosis drugs. There is also Frank Ryan's racy *Tuberculosis: The Greatest Story Never Told* (Bromsgrove: Swift Publishers, 1992).

On mass radiography, in addition to the papers referred to in the endnotes for this chapter, see the paper by A. L. Cochrane, 'The detection of pulmonary tuberculosis in a community', *British Medical Bulletin*, 10/2 (1954), 91–5 (part of a special issue on tuberculosis), reviewing the costs and benefits of this work, and Joint Tuberculosis Council, 'Review of mass radiography services', *Tubercle*, 45 (1964), 255–66. J. E. Golub et al., 'Active case finding of tuberculosis: historical perspective and future prospects', *International Journal of Lung Disease*, 9/11 (2005), 1183–203 is a recent update of the same kinds of issues. Watch a Pathé News recording from Glasgow at <http://www.youtube.com/watch?v=21_ddVcx94s> accessed 16 May 2012. Useful on the history of the mass X-ray campaign are Peter J. Tyler, *No Charge, No Undressing: Fronting Up for Good Health* (Sydney: Community Health and Tuberculosis Australia, 2003) for Australia, and Anne Hardy, 'Reframing disease: changing perceptions of tuberculosis in England and Wales, 1938–90', *Historical Research*, 76/194 (2003), 535–56 for the UK.

For the (now legendary) British trial of streptomycin see Alan Yoshioka, 'Use of randomisation in the Medical Research Council's clinical trial of streptomycin in pulmonary tuberculosis in the 1940s', *British Medical Journal*, 317 (1998), 1220–3 and John Crofton, 'The MRC randomized trial of streptomycin and its legacy: a view from the clinical front line', *Journal of the Royal Society of Medicine*, 99 (2006), 531–4. Yoshioka continues the drug's story in 'Streptomycin in postwar Britain: a cultural history of a miracle drug', in M. Gijswijt-Hofstra et al. (eds.), *Biographies of Remedies: Drugs, Medicines and Contraceptives in Dutch and Anglo-American Healing Cultures* (Amsterdam: Rodopi, 2002).

See also Helen Valier, 'At home in the colonies: the WHO–MRC trials at the Madras Chemotherapy Centre in the 1950s and 1960s', in Flurin Condrau and Michael Worboys (eds.), *Tuberculosis Then and Now* (Montreal and Kingston: McGill-Queens University Press, 2010), pp. 213–34, and Sunil Amrith, 'Plague of poverty: the World Health Organization, tuberculosis and international development, c.1945–1980' (M.Phil. thesis, University of Cambridge, 2002) and 'In search of a magic bullet for tuberculosis: south India and beyond, *c.*1955–1965', *Social History of Medicine*, 17/1 (2004), 113–30. For trials involving the Navajo see David Jones, 'The health care experiments at many farms: the Navajo, tuberculosis and the limits of modern medicine, 1951–1962', *Bulletin of the History of Medicine*, 76/4 (2002), 749–90. A witness seminar, D. A. Christie and E. M. Tansey (eds.), *Short-Course Chemotherapy for Tuberculosis* (London: Wellcome Trust, 2005), reviewed much of the research into treatment protocols and provides a useful bibliography. In Wallace Fox, 'The chemotherapy and epidemiology of tuberculosis: some findings of general applicability from the Tuberculosis Chemotherapy Centre, Madras', *The Lancet*, 280 (1962), 413–17, 473–8, one of the leaders discusses his results from Madras. M. C. Raviglione and A. Pio, 'Evolution of WHO policies for tuberculosis control, 1948–2001', *The Lancet*, 359 (2002), 775–80 is a useful insider's survey.

Chapter 9

Two excellent collections of essays by historians and those working in the field are Matthew Gandy and Alimuddin Zumla, *The Return of the White Plague: Global Poverty and the 'New' Tuberculosis* (London: Verso, 2003) and Condrau and Worboys (eds.), *Tuberculosis Then and Now*.

On immigrants and refugees see the work of John Welshman, 'Tuberculosis and ethnicity in England and Wales, 1950–70', *Sociology of Health & Illness*, 22/6 (2000), 858–82 and 'Importation, deprivation, and susceptibility: tuberculosis narratives in postwar Britain', in Condrau and Worboys (eds.), *Tuberculosis Then and Now*, pp. 123–47; Alison Bashford, 'The Great White Plague turns alien: tuberculosis and immigration in Australia, 1901–2001', in Condrau and Worboys (eds.), *Tuberculosis Then and Now*, pp. 100–22; Nicholas B. King, 'Immigration, race and geographies of difference in the tuberculosis pandemic', in Gandy and Zumla (eds.), *The Return of the White Plague*, pp. 39–54; Matthew Smallman-Raynor and Andrew D. Cliff, 'War and disease: some perspectives on the spatial and temporal occurrence of tuberculosis in wartime', in Gandy and Zumla (eds.), *The Return of the White Plague*, pp. 70–95; H. L. Rieder et al., 'Tuberculosis control in refugee settlements', *Tubercle*, 70 (1989), 127–34; and Rieder et al., 'Tuberculosis control in Europe and international migration', *European Respiratory Journal*, 7 (1994), 1545–53; and the very useful summary by John Porter and Claudia Kessler, 'Tuberculosis in refugees: a neglected dimension of the "global epidemic of tuberculosis"', *Transactions of the Royal Society of Tropical Medicine & Hygiene*, 89 (1995), 241–2.

Barron H. Lerner, *Contagion and Confinement: Controlling Tuberculosis along the Skid Road* (Baltimore: Johns Hopkins University Press, 1998) provides valuable insights on tuberculosis and the underclass of Seattle. Richard J. Coker, *From Chaos to Coercion: Detention and the Control of Tuberculosis* (New York: St Martin's Press, 2000) carries the story forward in New York in some pithy prose. I relied too upon the fine chapters by Deborah Wallace and Roderick Wallace, 'The recent tuberculosis epidemic in New York City: warning from the de-developing world', in Gandy and Zumla (eds.), *The Return of the White Plague*, pp. 125–46 and David S. Barnes, 'Targeting patient zero', in Condrau and Worboys (eds.), *Tuberculosis Then and Now*, pp. 49–71. Lee B. Reichman with Janice Hopkins Tanne, *Timebomb: The Global Epidemic of Multi-Drug Resistant Tuberulcois* (New York: McGraw-Hill, 2002) offers a dramatic insider's account of drug-resistant tuberculosis in New York and Russia. For the latter country see also Vivien Stern, 'The House of the Dead revisited: prisons, tuberculosis and public health in the former Soviet bloc', in Gandy and Zumla (eds.), *The Return of the White Plague*, pp. 178–94. The special issue of the *Journal of Law, Medicine & Ethics*, 21/3–4 (1993) contains a series of excellent papers on the history and contemporary problems of tuberculosis and HIV/AIDS.

Useful primary sources besides those in the chapter endnotes that helped reconstruct the DOTS and Stop TB stories are M. C. Raviglione et al., 'Secular trends of tuberculosis in western Europe', *Bulletin of the World Health Organization*, 71/3–4 (1993), 297–306; Ronald Bayer and David Wilkinson, 'Directly observed therapy for tuberculosis: history of an idea', *The Lancet*, 345 (1995),

1545–8; Mario C. Raviglione et al., 'Assessment of worldwide tuberculosis control', *The Lancet*, 350 (1997), 624–9; Ariel Pablos-Méndez et al., 'Global surveillance for antituberculosis-drug resistance', *New England Journal of Medicine*, 338/23 (1998), 1641–9; T. R. Friedman et al., 'Lessons from the 1800s: tuberculosis control in the new millennium', *The Lancet*, 355 (2000), 1088–92; A. M. C. Rose et al., 'Tuberculosis at the end of the 20th century in England and Wales: results of a national survey in 1998', *Thorax*, 56 (2001), 173–9; John A. Sbarbaro, 'Kochi's tuberculosis strategy article is a "classic" by any definition', *Bulletin of the World Health Organization*, 79/1 (2001), 69–75, which includes a reprint of Kochi's article from 1991, 'The global tuberculosis situation and the new control of strategy of the World Health Organization'; T. Arnadottir, 'The styblo model 20 years later: what holds true?', *International Journal of Tuberculosis and Lung Disease*, 13/6 (2009), 672–90; T. Arnadottir, *Tuberculosis and Public Health: Policy and Principles in Tuberculosis Control* (Paris: International Union against Tuberculosis and Lung Disease, 2009); Paul Farmer and Jim Yong Kim, 'Community based approaches to the control of multidrug-resistant tuberculosis: introducing "DOTS-plus"', *British Medical Journal*, 317 (1998), 671–4; Paul Farmer and David Walton, 'The social impact of multi-drug resistant tuberculosis: Haiti and Peru', in Gandy and Zumla (eds.), *The Return of the White Plague*, pp. 163–77.

Epilogue

Paul Mayho, *The Tuberculosis Survival Handbook* (London: XLR8, 1988) is Mayho's diary cum self-help manual. Antony Alpers, *The Life of Katherine Mansfield* (Harmondsworth: Penguin, 1982) is one of several biographies of Mansfield; see also C. A. Hankin (ed.), *The Letters of John Middleton Murry to Katherine Mansfield* (Auckland: Hutchinson, 1983).

For the latest WHO report on tuberculosis see 'WHO warns of consequences of underfunding TB', <http://www.who.int/mediacentre/news/releases/2011/tb_20111011/en/> accessed 16 May 2012.

INDEX

Note: page numbers in *italic* refer to illustrations.

open-air cure 134, 135 136–40
operas 91–3
opium/opiates 49, 66, 97
Orwell, George: xiii–xvi,
    xix–xxii, xxiii–xxvii,
    xxviii, 58
O'Shaughnessy, Eileen: xvi,
    xxi–xxii
O'Shaughnessy, Laurence: xvi, xxii
osteomyelitis 2
outpatient treatment
    India 217–21
    pneumothorax refills 152
    USA 241
    see also dispensaries

Paimio Sanatorium, Finland 128
palaeopathology 5
palaeosteology 5–6
Papier d'Arménie 120
Papua New Guinea 237
para-aminosalicylic acid, see PAS
Park, William Hallock 181
Parker's Tonic 109
Partners in Health (PIH) 263, 264
PAS (para-aminosalicylic acid)
    xxvi, 197–9, 219
Pasteur, Louis 105, 190, 191
Paterson, Marcus 142–3
patient experiences
    Brontë sisters 88–90
    Clark, Alice 141–2
    Keats, John 79–81
    Keats, Tom 79
    MacDonald, Betty 143–5,
        154, 157
    Mansfield, Katherine 268
    Mayho, Paul 268
    a merchant, 68
    Orwell, George: xiii–xvi,
        xix–xxii, xxiii–xxvii
    sanatorium life 128, 130, 131,
        136, 137–46, 163–6, 194

Smollett, Tobias 69–70, 73
    Violetta 91–3
    Wagstaffe, Peter 165
PCR (polymerase chain reaction)
    amplification 7–8
pectorals 48, 65
pectoriloquy 58
People's Union of the Red
    Cross 132–3
PEPFAR (President's Emergency
    Plan for Aids Relief) 266
Peruvian balsam 65, 66
Pfuhl, Eduard 147
Pharnunches 15
Philip, Robert 115–17, 120, 151
Philips electrical industries,
    Australia 204–5
phrenicectomy 156
phrenicotomy 156–7
Phthisiologia (Morton) 45
phthisics 15, 21
phthisis 10–22, 54–6
    predisposition to 15–16
    spread of 21–2
    treatment of 18–21
    tubercles in 17–18
    types of 14–15, 16
    see also consumption;
        tuberculosis
physiology: knowledge of 31
Piave, Francesco Maria 91
PIH (Partners in Health) 263, 264
Piorkowski, Dr 149
Plague and I, The (MacDonald)
    143–4
pleural shock 155
Pneumatic Institute, Hotwells
    73, 74
Pneumocystis carinii
    pneumonia 244
pneumonectomy 159
pneumoperitoneum
    156, 157